Dear Scott

It is always

a pleasure to

see you.

Best wishes

Caroline

Beiträge zum Gesundheitsmanagement

Herausgeber:
Prof. Dr. rer. oec. Norbert Klusen
Andreas Meusch

Band 32

Norbert Klusen/Frank Verheyen/
Caroline Wagner (eds.)

England and Germany in Europe – What Lessons Can We Learn from Each Other?

European Health Care Conference 2011

 Nomos

Die Deutsche Nationalbibliothek verzeichnet diese Publikation in
der Deutschen Nationalbibliografie; detaillierte bibliografische
Daten sind im Internet über http://dnb.d-nb.de abrufbar.

Die Deutsche Nationalbibliothek lists this publication in the
Deutsche Nationalbibliografie; detailed bibliographic data
is available in the Internet at http://dnb.d-nb.de.

ISBN 978-3-8329-6704-8

1. Auflage 2011
© Nomos Verlagsgesellschaft, Baden-Baden 2011. Printed in Germany. Alle Rechte,
auch die des Nachdrucks von Auszügen, der fotomechanischen Wiedergabe und der
Übersetzung, vorbehalten. Gedruckt auf alterungsbeständigem Papier.

Preface

These days Germany and all other EU member states face difficult economic times and crucial health policy changes – at national as well as at European level. There is a growing need to share experiences and ideas across borders – also between health systems. This is why we decided that we as the Scientific Institute of Techniker Krankenkasse for Benefit and Efficiency in Health Care (WINEG) and Techniker Krankenkasse (TK) will host the second European Health Care Conference 2011 in cooperation with the European Health Management Association (EHMA) from Brussels on 20 May here at our headquarters in Hamburg.

After a period of intensive expertise interchange with e.g. the English National Health Service (NHS), the Department of Health and The Nuffield Trust in London, we realised how different the situation in health care is in Germany, but at the same time how similar in some aspects the challenges are. In consequence, this time the conference will compare health care in England to health care in Germany and consider the impact of European health policy on them: »England and Germany in Europe – What lessons can we learn from each other?« In other words: if Bismarck and Beveridge had met, what would they have learned from each other? And what would they have thought about the European development in health care?

The purpose behind this imaginative picture is to synthesize expert observations about approaches of fund allocation and of health services provision in the English National Health Service (NHS) which could improve the quality and efficiency in German health care – and vice versa. For this we were able to gain experts from health policy, health academia and health management to discuss the future of the English NHS – particularly the ongoing health care reform – and the German statutory health insurance. We are delighted that most of them – despite the time restrictions of their busy diaries – were able to contribute to this conference publication with a paper elaborating in more depth the theses of their presentations at our conference.

In contrast, three years ago, at our first European Health Care Conference in cooperation with EHMA, we focused on a variety of EU health systems instead of two. Nearly 300 participants from 19 countries (including non-European countries like the US, Mexico, Russia and Nigeria) had the opportunity to follow the inspiring debate of leading experts from academia and from the field in the US, the UK, the Netherlands, Italy, Austria, the Czech Republic and Germany.

The one-day conference reflected about »The Future of European Health Care Systems« and thus fostered the sharing of knowledge about health policy issues between these six EU member states and the US. Moreover we sought to generate a platform for the international discussion of the considerable changes in German health care caused by the health care reform in 2009.

The feedback was excellent: the speakers, the participants and the press perceived the conference as an important contribution to the national and international health policy debate. Thus the conference was appraised as a great success. Moreover the new findings enabled us to give German and European health policy fresh impetus on behalf of our insurants.

TK and its WINEG will definitely benefit from the findings and other impulses that this Anglo-German dialogue in health care across the channel generates. A selection of these sophisticated analyses and inspiring thoughts is gathered in this conference publication. Enjoy reading!

Professor Dr *Norbert Klusen*
Chairman of the Board of Management of Techniker Krankenkasse

Dr *Frank Verheyen*
Director of the Scientific Institute of TK for Benefit
and Efficiency in Health Care (WINEG)

Table of Contents

Chapter 1:
Health Care in England, Germany and Europe:
Potential for Future Reforms?

Adoption of a Cost-Saving Innovation: Germany, UK and Simvastatin

Thomas G. McGuire, Sebastian Bauhoff

Abstract

We examine how the UK and German health care systems responded to a major cost-saving innovation: the availability of generic simvastatin, a cholesterol-lowering drug. In the German Social Health Insurance, the generic's entry reduced sales volumes for both branded simvastatin (Zocor) and a close substitute, branded atorvastatin (Lipitor/Sortis). In UK, only the sales of branded simvastatin fell whereas the sales of atorvastatin were mostly unaffected. We trace these experiences to institutional differences in the two health care systems and to the structure of patient cost-sharing in particular.

Zusammenfassung

Wir untersuchen die Reaktionen des britischen und des deutschen Gesundheitssystems auf eine der bedeutendsten kostensparenden Innovationen: die Verfügbarkeit von generischem Simvastatin, einem cholesterinsenkenden Medikament. Die Zulassung des Generikums senkte bei den gesetzlichen Krankenkassen in Deutschland die Verkaufsvolumen sowohl bei dem Markenprodukt Simvastatin (Zocor) als auch bei einem sehr ähnlichen Ersatzwirkstoff, dem Markenprodukt Atorvastatin (Lipitor/Sortis). In Großbritannien führte die Zulassung nur bei dem Markenprodukt Simvastatin zu geringeren Verkaufszahlen, wohingegen der Verkauf von Atorvastatin kaum betroffen war. Wir führen dies auf institutionelle Unterschiede beider Gesundheitssysteme und besonders auf die Struktur der Kostenbeteiligung des Patienten zurück.

Introduction

Health care systems can be compared in terms of costs (spending per capita, share of GDP devoted to health care, spending growth), outcomes (longevity, maternal death rates), and fairness (solidarity in financing, disparities in services), all system metrics determined by many factors. Working with such aggregates has some limitations. A finding, for example, that Germany spends more per capita than the UK on health care, calls attention to an issue, but, by itself, has no direct implication for health policy. Furthermore, an overall measure, like spending, averages many activities. It is unlikely, comparing two health care systems, that one will be superior to another in all components of the average. For identification and exchange of productive approaches – for mutual learning – specific comparisons are more likely to uncover instances where one system solves a problem more effectively than another.

This paper compares the German and UK health care systems as they respond to a particular cost-saving innovation: the availability in 2004 of the generic statin simvastatin, previously sold as Merck's branded Zocor. Statins, a widely used and effective class of cholesterol-reducing drugs, were developed based on research on cholesterol synthesis at the Max Planck Institute in the 1950s. Statin drugs, while effective, are costly to health payers. In 2004, another branded statin, Lipitor (atorvastatin, sold as Sortis in Germany) was the largest selling drug, with worldwide sales of US $ 12.0 bn; in the same year, Zocor was the second-largest selling drug with sales of US $ 5.9 bn (OFT 2007: 39).

Simvastatin was the first widely used statin to be available as a generic. How did the health care systems in Germany and the UK respond to this opportunity? Specifically, how quickly was the generic version available in each country? At what price to the national health system (and to consumers)? How rapidly did simvastatin displace Zocor? Finally, and here is where Germany and UK will diverge the most: to what degree did simvastatin substitute for Lipitor?

In the following sections we first outline the coverage and pricing practices for pharmaceuticals in Germany and the UK.[1] We highlight key differences between the systems in the managing of generic entry with regards to regulatory processes and consequences for the patented drug. We then turn to the experience with generic simvastatin, which had large impacts on an important segment of the prescription drug market in both countries. The differential impact in Germany and the UK reflects the regulatory and institutional variations that underlie the adoption of cost-saving technology in these contexts.

Drug review, coverage and pricing

German Social Health Insurance

In the German Social Health Insurance (SHI), coverage and pricing decisions are made by a joint federal committee (Gemeinsamer Bundesaus-

---

1   Kanavos, Costa-Font and McGuire (2007) compare the markets for and regulation of drug policies in UK, Germany, Netherlands and France in relation to branded statin products over the period 1991–2002.

schuss).[2] Most covered drugs are subject to reference pricing, whereby the joint committee determines the drug groupings and the reference price as maximum reimbursement through the funds.[3] There are three forms of reference groups, depending on the included drugs. The reference price is set within the lower third of the included drugs' market prices since 2006; at least a fifth of prescriptions and packages must be at or below the reference price (§ 35 SGB V). In addition to the SHI-wide reference price, individual funds can negotiate rebates with manufacturers in exchange for exclusivity in generic supply.

Until recently, manufacturers were free to set the prices for new, patented drugs. The November 2010 health reform (Arzneimittelmarktneuordnungsgesetz, in effect since January 2011) constrains the price-setting ability depending on whether a new molecule provides additional benefits. Under the new regulations manufacturers remain free to set initial prices. However, this price is revisited in the first 3-12 months as the joint committee assesses whether the drug provides benefits relative to existing treatments. If the committee recognizes no additional benefit, the reference price applies. If the manufacturer can demonstrate additional benefits, the firm and sickness funds (as a group) negotiate a reimbursable price. An independent arbiter will determine a price if the funds and manufacturer do not come to a resolution within 12 months.

Physicians are only subject to weak incentives regarding pharmaceuticals. Physician associations and sickness funds agree on regional targets for pharmaceutical expenditures, which are then applied to individual practices. In principle, practices were responsible for costs exceeding prescribing budgets yet these fines have rarely been imposed (Brandt, 2008; Kanavos et al., 2008). An additional but short-lived *bonus-malus* rule for specific groups of drugs created financial incentives for individual physicians to limit (over-) prescribing. However, this rule was abolished in the 2010 reforms (BMG, 2010).

Pharmacies play a central role in the German system. First, they are responsible for collecting copayments, which are described below. Second, pharmacists are required to substitute toward cheaper drugs with the same chemical, concentration and package size, unless the prescription precludes substitution (*aut idem* rule). Pharmacies are also responsible for dispensing according to any rebate contracts that individual funds may have negotiated with generic manufacturers.

---

2   The committee consists of physician, dentist, hospital and sickness fund representatives. In this section we focus on outpatient prescribing.
3   The distribution via wholesale and pharmacies adds an additional cost to pharmaceuticals. Both institutions receive a regulated flat fee and percentage of the drug's price. Manufacturers must offer a mandatory discount to all sickness funds; this discount has been temporarily modified several times.

Finally, patients are subject to copayments of 10 per cent of the sales price and between 5 and 10 Euro per prescription; this copayment is transferred to the sickness funds.[4] The sales price is the price paid by consumers in the pharmacy and consists of the manufacturer's price plus margins for wholesalers and the pharmacy. In cases where the reference price applies, patients are also responsible for any costs beyond this price: since the reference price determines the reimbursement by the sickness funds, patients must self-finance the difference between the reference and sales prices. Conversely, all copayments are waived for drugs that are at least 30 per cent below the reference price. Copays may also be reduced for medications purchased under a rebate contract. Because the reference price plays an important part in determining patient copays, physicians must inform patients when prescribing a drug that is priced above the reference price.

Table 1 illustrates the current structure of patient copayments for Lipitor, and branded and generic simvastatin in Germany. These drugs are subject to the same reference price but have substantially different sales prices. In particular, Lipitor is priced substantially above the reference price, leading to high patient copays. The generic simvastatin hits the floor of the statutory copay of 5 Euro.

Table 1: *Example of copayments for selected statins (Euro)*

	Sortis / Lipitor (Atorvastatin)	Zocor (Simvastatin)	Generic (Simvastatin)
Sales price	57.36	22.66	13.34
Reference price	13.36	13.36	13.36
Diff. sales – reference price, if positive	44	9.30	n/a
Regular copay	5 (min copay)	5 (min copay)	5 (min copay)
Total patient copay	49	14.30	5

Notes: example for fourth quarter of 2010 and package of 30 film tables of 20 mg active ingredient. The generic simvastatin is produced by ratiopharm. Prices from DIMDI, 2010.

4   Children below the age of 18 are exempt from these copays, and pharmaceutical expenditures count toward an income-related cap on total out-of-pocket costs.

United Kingdom National Health Service

The UK National Health Service (NHS) uses separate pricing schemes for branded and generic drugs. The Pharmaceutical Price Regulation Scheme (PPRS) applies to patented drugs. The Scheme determines list prices indirectly by setting profitability and is negotiated between the Department of Health and the pharmaceutical industry association for a period of about five years. Manufacturers are free to set initial prices for New Active Substances but subsequent price increases are subject to approval.[5] In practice, these price controls are more binding than the profit controls (OFT, 2007).

Reimbursement rates for generics under the Drugs Tariff are based on volume-weighted average ex-factory prices across available generics in the UK. Since the amount paid to the pharmacy is not tied to the pharmacy's actual cost, this procedure has led to sharp declines in generic prices: in 2005, the average annual decrease in generic prices in the UK was nearly five times higher than in Germany (32.4 and 6.9 per cent respectively; see OFT, 2007-A: 62).

As in Germany there are weak controls on prescribing at the physician-level. While the National Institute for Clinical Excellence (NICE) offers guidelines that include considerations for cost effectiveness and the British National Formulary points to generic prescribing for each drug entry, GPs are free to choose among therapeutically equivalent medicines. Moreover, financial incentives for GPs to prescribe cost-effective medications are limited: the key contracting arrangements are between the Primary Care Organisations (PCO) and GP practices rather than individual physicians, and the contract specifies mostly clinical targets that may not align with cost-containment considerations (OFT, 2007-A). PCOs may use local incentive structures to manage prescribing, but overall GPs have been found to »have weak knowledge of the prices of some of the most widely-prescribed drugs in the UK« (OFT, 2007: 2) and are presumed to be relatively insensitive to drug prices in their prescribing decisions.[6]

Prescriptions are issued for a specific brand or written generically using the chemical's name, and dispensing and reimbursements at the pharmacy-level vary accordingly. When the physician explicitly prescribes the brand, or when the physician writes the chemical and no generic is available, pharmacists

---

5   The profit and price controls apply at the level of the manufacturer rather than specific drugs. The PPRS updates may include temporary, across-the-board price cuts. Manufacturers can »modulate« prices of individual drugs in their portfolio to achieve these savings. The repeated use of these cuts has led to concerns about strategic behaviour by manufacturers as they anticipate future adjustments (e.g. OFT, 2007).

6   The practice-level incentive schemes and, from 2004, the Quality Outcomes Framework may have increased price sensitivity, but the available evidence is mixed (Walley et al., 2005).

must dispense the brand and the associated reimbursement is based on manufacturers' list prices as governed by the PPRS.[7] For a generically written prescription the reimbursement is based on the average price of generics in the market plus a dispensing margin which represents a financing arrangement between the NHS and pharmacies.[8] The two parallel approaches to determining reimbursements imply that dispensing margins on generics are higher than margins on branded drugs.

Patients contribute flat-fee copayments (of £ 7.40 in England as of 1 April 2001) for medication purchases, the same for brand or generics. Many exemptions (young, old, unemployed) imply that the majority of prescriptions are free. Overall patients in England pay only 5.6 per cent of drug costs (OFT, 2007: 14).

Table 2 summarises the key features from this and the previous section. Overall the pricing for generics in the UK is more aggressive than in Germany since it is constructed as volume-weighted average, and pharmacies have a strong incentive to shop for the lowest cost source. The default substitution in the pharmacy and variable patient copayments in Germany imply there is likely to be a greater response to high manufacturer prices for a brand in the presence of generic alternatives.[9]

---

7   The reimbursements are based on predetermined price schedules (list and ex-factory prices) rather than actual prices paid, so that pharmacies have incentives to procure from the cheapest source, including parallel imports. Since pharmacies may receive discounts from manufacturers of branded and generic drugs, the NHS shares potential profits through a variable clawback payment (the average payment is 9.2 per cent of total monthly reimbursements; OFT, 2007: 30). The clawback creates a wedge between the list price and actual reimbursement.

8   As procurement agents for PCOs, pharmacies receive a guaranteed level of income that is operationalised through contractual dispensing margins. This retained profit margin is achieved mainly through manipulation of the reimbursement rates of generics in Category M of the Drugs Tariff (OFT, 2007: 32; OFT, 2007-A: 52).

9   The Office of Fair Trading (OFT, 2007: 15) was critical of incentives to substitute in the UK. »As these brief descriptions suggest, demand for drugs within the NHS (particularly in primary care) is characterised by a complex set of principal-agent relationships, in which:
    •   the person who consumes the drug (the patient) neither decides nor, in most cases, pays
    •   the person who decides which drug should be used (the prescribing doctor) neither pays nor consumes, and
    •   the institution that pays for the drug (the NHS / Government) neither consumes nor decides.«

Table 2: *Key features of pharmaceutical policies in the UK and Germany*

	UK	Germany
Supply-side measures		
Generic firms allowed to complete regulatory requirements prior to patent expiry (Bolar provisions)	Y	Y
Price cap	Y	
Reference pricing		Y
Proxy demand-side policies		
Promoting generic prescribing	Y	Y
Compulsory generic prescribing		
Prescribing monitoring and audit	Y	Y
Default generic substitution at pharmacy		Y
Flat fee combined with regressive margin for pharmacy		Y
Flat fee for pharmacy		
Discounting allowed for pharmacy	Y	
Clawback of pharmacy profits	Y	
Demand-side policies		
Differential co-payments		Y
Flat fee	Y	

Source: based on Kanavos (2008) and Kanavos et al. (2008), with modifications, Y = yes

Managing generic entry in Germany and the UK

How do the German and the UK institutions outlined above handle the introduction of a generic drug? In Germany, the entrant would fall into a reference group with an associated price that represents the maximum reimbursable cost for sickness funds. Individual sickness funds could negotiate rebate contracts with the manufacturer, triggering default substitution in the pharmacy and lower copayments for their patients. Physicians must inform patients if a prescribed drug is priced above the reference price and hence generates higher patient copays. As a result, physicians may be price responsive agents for patients who are at risk for cost-sharing.[10]

In the UK, the generic would be priced under the Drug Tariff, i.e. as a function of ex-factory prices and market shares of other generics. GPs are not required to switch patients to the cheaper medication. Any updates in prescribing guidelines by NICE are not binding and the financial incentives to substitute are weak for individual physicians. Substitution yields no savings in copayments for patients that could outweigh any transaction costs from switching.[11] As consequence, there is little cause to switch patients to the generic, or to write the prescription with the chemical's name so as to allow substitution in the pharmacy. The potentially rapid decline in generic prices under the Drug Tariff's pricing formula increases pharmacy margins for generics but are not transmitted to either physicians or patients.

A comparative perspective from the United States

In the US, drug coverage and pricing is decentralised to private managed care plans and public purchasers. Most private payers use three-tier formularies, with generic drugs on the first tier requiring a small copayment from the patient, »preferred brand« drugs on the second tier requiring a moderate copayment, and other branded drugs on the third tier requiring the highest copayment (KFF, 2009).[12]

A drug formulary encourages use of lower-priced generics when these are available, and more generally, encourages, by favourable tier placement, medications which the plan regards to be more cost-effective (Grabowski and Mullins, 1997). A formulary also puts a plan in good bargaining position with manufacturers, especially in the presence of therapeutic alternatives among branded drugs for treating particular conditions. Plans do not put all drugs for some conditions on the formulary. By choosing the drug or drugs for favourable formulary placement, the plan can offer a manufacturer favourable tier placement – which translates into higher sales volume – in exchange for rebates (Huskamp et al., 2003; Grabowski and Mullins, 1997; Frank, 2001).[13]

A typical drug formulary in a managed care plan covers only some of the many available statins. Duggan et al. (2008: 77-78) examined the inclusion on

---

10 Direct-to-consumer advertising of prescription drugs is not allowed in Germany, possibly further increasing the cross-price elasticity.
11 In addition, the different approaches for pricing branded and generic drugs (particularly the dispensing margins) can mitigate the price differential from the GP perspective.
12 Danzon and Ketcham (2004) discuss differences between formularies and therapeutic reference pricing.
13 Huskamp et al. (2003: 154) find savings of about 30 per cent by the Veterans' Administration when it established closed classes in its national formulary.

formularies of 20 of the top-selling brand name statin drugs in three large private Part D plans serving Medicare beneficiaries in California in 2007.

»The formulary status and prices of each drug vary substantially across plans. In the AARP plan, for example, five of the 20 drugs were preferred, eight were non-preferred, and the other seven were off-formulary [no coverage]. In the WellCare plan, three were preferred, on nonpreferred, and 16 off-formulary. In the Sierra plan, four were preferred and 16 were off-formulary ... There was little overlap between these plans in formulary placement; for example, only one drug (Zetia) was on the preferred tier in all three plans. This latter finding suggests that statin manufacturers were selective in providing discounts to these plans in exchange for better (or exclusive) formulary placement.«

Generic drugs, like simvastatin, are always first-tier in formularies. (One of the authors of this paper gets his 90-day supply of simvastatin by mail for a US $ 15 copay.)[14]

Once a generic version of a drug becomes available in the US, state-level regulations lead to aggressive and immediate substitution for the brand. Even if the physician writes »Zocor« on the prescription, pharmacies dispense a generic. Formulary coverage policies reinforce the substitution, so that within about two months of generic entry, brand sales fall to less than 10 per cent of the pre-generic level.[15]

Simvastatin experience

Statins are a major drug class of cholesterol-reducing medications and include a variety of active ingredients, most importantly in terms of sales, atorvastatin and simvastatin. Atorvastatin is still under patent by Pfizer and sold under the brand name of Lipitor (Sortis in Germany). Simvastatin is the active ingredi-

---

14 The website for Medco (a pharmacy benefit manager) for Harvard employees indicates that the branded statins on Tier 2 are Lescol, Lipitor, Altoprev, Livalo, Crestor, Mevacor and Pravachol. Comparing Simvastatin and Liptior, the website reports:

	Annual Costs		
	You pay	Plan Pays	Total
Simvastatin	$60	$168.71	$228.71
Lipitor	$140	$1445.04	$1585.04

There is also the following disclaimer: »The cost that is displayed, however, does not include any additional discount or other incentives your plan may receive from your use of this medication.«

15 For a recent review, see Berndt and Newhouse (2010). The drug patent regulations in the US were reformed in 1984, extending in some cases patent life for new drugs, but encouraging generic entry and legal challenges to patents. The upshot is that in some cases drugs go off patent in the US later than in other countries. This was true for Zocor which did not have generic competition in the US until 2006. Berndt and Newhouse (2010) also discuss US patent policy.

ent in Zocor, a product of Merck. When used in their standard dosage, atorvastatin and simvastatin have similar clinical outcomes (e.g., Zhou et al., 2006) and are considered close substitutes for the majority of patients. Statins represent a large share of prescription drug expenditures worldwide.

The expiration of Merck's patent on simvastatin in May 2003 in Germany and the UK, and the subsequent emergence of generic simvastatin were associated with large shifts in the prices and use of statins in both countries. Generic simvastatin provides a useful case study of a potentially disruptive cost-saving technology that the German and UK institutions translated into different outcomes for the health systems. In this section we chronicle the impact of generic simvastatin on the branded Zocor and the therapeutic substitute Lipitor.[16] While generic simvastatin led to a precipitous drop in market share for Lipitor in Germany, it did not have corresponding impact on Lipitor sales in the UK. The market share of Zocor declined steeply in both countries as generic competitors entered. We trace these experiences to institutional differences in the two health care systems.

Prices and market shares

Zocor lost patent protection in Germany in May 2003, leading to the immediate entry of generic producers and a rapid switch from branded to generic simvastatin.[17] This may be due to the *aut idem* substitution in the pharmacy, which encourages lower-priced products.

In addition, the expiration of Zocor's patent impacted the market for its close but patented substitute, Lipitor. The joint federal committee created a single reference group for all statins in 2004, with a common reference price from January 2005. The reference group includes drugs that are on-patent and therapeutically similar, making Lipitor subject to the reimbursement ceiling. Pfizer mounted a legal challenge against the application of the reference price but lost in the first and appeals instances (G-BA, 2010).

Figure 1 shows the evolution of market shares by molecule in the German statin market before and after the introduction of the reference pricing in January 2005. Despite the significant gap between the sales and reference prices for Lipitor, Pfizer did not reduce Lipitor's price, leading to a significant

---

16   Throughout we compare atorvastatin and simvastatin of similar package sizes, delivery modes and strength. Although the potency of these two ingredients differs somewhat, we adopt OFT's (2007-A: 41) view that adjusting for potency does not lead to different substantive conclusions because of the very large price differences.

17   Prior to patent expiration, Merck introduced its own »fighter brand« Zocor MSD and sold early-entry rights to a generics producer. As result, the market share of branded Zocor started declining from early 2003 (Raasch, 2006).

increase in patient copayments for Lipitor. The consequence was a sharp drop in Lipitor's market share from the second half of 2004 to the first half of 2005, mostly to the benefit of simvastatin. Lipitor maintained its market share in the private health insurance, which was not subject to the copay shock.

Figure 1: *Market share of statins before and after reference pricing in Jan 2005*

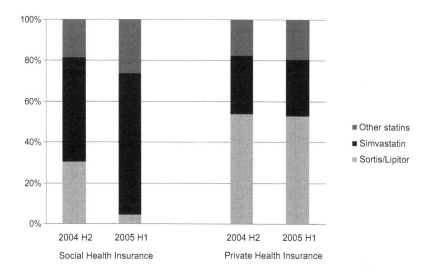

Notes: H1 and H2 refer to the first and second half of the year, respectively. Reference pricing is only used in social health insurance. Adapted from Wild (2006).

Merck's patent on simvastatin in the UK also expired in May 2003, leading to entry and a rapid decrease in prices for generic simvastatin (Figure 2a). In this context, the substitution was almost entirely from Zocor to generic simvastatin: Figure 2b shows that the decrease in sales for Zocor is recovered by its generic competitors. Lipitor's sales trend remains unaffected, indicating the lack of switching away from the on-patent statins despite a very substantial price advantage. This strikingly low cross-price elasticity has raised concerns over foregone savings to the NHS (OFT, 2007).

Figure 2a: *Prices of selected statins in the UK*

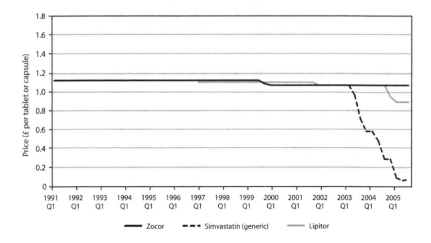

Notes: Tablets with 20mg active ingredient; adapted from OFT (2007).

Figure 2b: Sales volume of selected statins in the UK

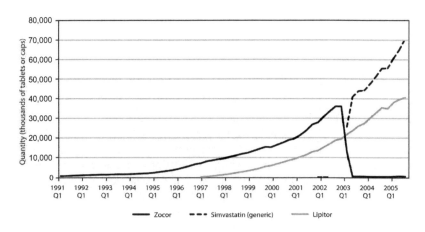

Notes: Tablets with 20mg active ingredient; adapted from OFT (2007).

Discussion

The impact of generic entry in Germany and the UK highlights how variations in health systems can affect outcomes. Both countries limit reimbursements as generics appear and encourage, but do not strictly require, physicians to prescribe such that pharmacists can substitute. The pharmacy-level substitution policies can explain the switch across drugs with the same molecule, i.e. from Zocor to generic simvastatin. In the German case, this substitution operates through the default *aut idem* requirement. In the UK, pharmacies may dispense generics when the prescriber indicated the chemical's name.

However, active intervention by physicians is required to switch patients across molecules, i.e. from the still-patented Lipitor to generic simvastatin. This suggests that prescribing behaviour is critical to the different experiences in Germany and the UK. German physicians may be more effective agents for their patients because of the impact of drug choice on copays. The flat copayment and many exemptions in the UK imply that price differences are not transmitted to patients and, indirectly, physicians. Officials in the UK are aware of the ineffectiveness of the NHS in transmitting incentives for substitution down to the level at which action can be taken:

> »Competition between manufacturers did not lead to significant reductions in the price of substitute products, such as the other statins. Moreover, these substitute products retained significant volume and market shares despite the very significant change in relative price following simvastatin going off patent. Given the very low prices at which generics are available, sustained prescribing of high-priced brands that may be therapeutic substitutes for many patients, raises potentially very significant concerns about the cost effectiveness of prescribing behaviour.«
> (OFT, 2007: 26).

Developments in the US statin market also suggest the importance of coverage policy and patient cost-sharing to encourage switching across molecules by physicians. Zocor lost patent protection in the US in June 2006, later than in Germany or the UK. With simvastatin available generically, formularies moved Lipitor to higher tiers.[18] One pharmacy benefit manager moved Lipitor to tier 3 in January 2006 in anticipation of generic simvastatin, and saw more than 40 per cent of patients switch from Lipitor to a lower-tier statin (Cox et al., 2007). Among those with copayment differences of $ 21 or more, 80 per cent switched.[19]

---

18   See Aitken et al. (2008). US state generic substitution laws do not apply to simvastatin-Lipitor substitution.
19   See also Sy et al. (2009) who find a 40 per cent switching from Lipitor in a group of physicians.

Such decentralised efforts at substitution aggregated to a major effect on statin sales. As Aitken et al. (2008) report, the loss of Zocor's protection led to a rapid displacement of the branded drug with generic simvastatin. Moreover, Lipitor sales fell by 12 per cent overall and 26 per cent for new prescriptions.

The expiration of Zocor's patent and the subsequent changes in Germany and the UK provide a useful case study to how these health care systems adapt to cost-saving innovations.[20] In this instance the potential cost saving was transmitted into incentives to decision-makers (physicians and patients) more effectively in the German than in the UK system. At least in the case of drugs, there is considerable patient cost-sharing in the German system with a mechanism to leverage physician agency and encourage substitution. This seems to be largely absent in the UK, leading to costly prescribing patterns and a slower adoption of lower-cost treatments.

References

Aitken, M., E. R. Berndt, and D. M. Cutler (2009). Prescription Drug Spending Trends In The United States: Looking Beyond The Turning Point. *Health Affairs* 28(1): w151-w160.

Berndt, E. and Newhouse, J. P. (2010). *Pricing and Reimbursement in U.S. Pharmaceutical Markets*. NBER Working Paper 16297. National Bureau of Economic Research.

Cox, E. R., A. Kulkarni, and R. Henderson (2007). Impact of Patient and Plan Design Factors on Switching to Preferred Statin Therapy. *Annals of Pharmacotherapy* 41(12): 1946–1953.

Danzon, P. and J. Ketcham (2004). Reference Pricing of Pharmaceuticals for Medicare: Evidence from Germany, the Netherlands, and New Zealand. *Forum for Health Economics & Policy* 7: 1-54.

DIMDI (2010). *Arzneimittel-Festbeträge vom 1.10.2010*. Deutsches Institut für medizinische Dokumentation und Information.

Mark Duggan, Patrick Healy, and Fiona Scott Morton (2008). Providing Prescription Drug Coverage to the Elderly: America's Experiment with Medicare Part D. *Journal of Economic Perspectives* 22(4): 69-92.

Frank, R. G. (2001). Prescription Drug Prices: Why Do Some Pay More Than Others Do? *Health Affairs* 20(2): 115-128.

G-BA. (2010). *Rechtsstreit um Sortis: G-BA auch in zweiter Instanz gegen Pfizer erfolgreich (Pressemitteilung 5. März 2010)*. Gemeinsamer Bundesausschuss.

Grabowski, H. and C. D. Mullins (1997). Pharmacy Benefit Management, Cost-effectiveness Analysis and Drug Formulary Decisions. *Social Science & Medicine* 45(4): 535-544.

---

20   OFT (2007: 25) concurs that the experience with Zocor is common in the UK, making it a good example for related innovations.

Huskamp, H. A., A. M. Epstein, and D. Blumenthal (2003). The Impact of a National Prescription Drug Formulary on Prices, Market Share, and Spending: Lessons for Medicare? *Health Affairs* 22(3): 149-158.

Huskamp, H. A., P. A. Deverka, A. M. Epstein, R. S. Epstein, K. A. McGuigan, and R. G. Frank (2003). The Effect of Incentive-based Formularies on Prescription-drug Utilization and Spending. *New England Journal of Medicine* 349(23): 2224-2232.

Kanavos, P. (2008). Generic policies: Rhetoric vs. Reality. *Euro Observer 10*(2).

Kanavos, P., J. Costa-Font, and A. McGuire (2007). Product Differentiation, Competition and Regulation of New Drugs: The Case of Statins in Four European Countries. *Managerial and Decision Economics* 28: 445-465.

Kanavos, P., J. Costa-Font, and E. Seeley (2008). Competition in Off-patent Drug Markets: Issues, Regulation and Evidence. *Economic Policy* 23(55): 499-544.

KFF (2009). *Employer Health Benefits: 2009 Annual Survey*. Kaiser Family Foundation.

OFT (2007). *Pharmaceutical Price Regulation Scheme*. UK Office of Fair Trading.

OFT (2007-A). *Pharmaceutical Price Regulation Scheme. Annexe A: Markets for Prescription Pharmaceuticals in the NHS*. UK Office of Fair Trading.

Sy, F. Z., H. M. Choe, D. M. Kennedy, C. J. Standiford, D. M. Parsons, K. D. Bruhnsen, J. G. Stevenson, and S. J. Bernstein (2009). Moving from A to Z: Successful Implementation of a Statin Switch Program by a Large Physician Group. *The American Journal of Managed Care* 15(4): 233-240.

Raasch, A. (2006). *Der Patentauslauf von Pharmazeutika als Herausforderung beim Management des Produktlebenszyklus: Strategische Optionen und ihre erfolgreiche Umsetzung in Marketing und Vertrieb*. DUV.

Walley, T., Mrazek, M., & Mossialos, E. (2005). Regulating Pharmaceutical Markets: Improving Efficiency and Controlling Costs in the UK. *The International Journal of Health Planning and Management, 20*(4): 375-398.

Wild, F. (2006). *Arzneimittelversorgung von Privatversicherten: Der Markt der Statine*. WIP-Diskussionspapier 4/06. Wissenschaftliches Institut der PKV.

Zhou, Z., E. Rahme, and L. Pilote (2006). Are Statins Created Equal? Evidence from Randomized Trials of Pravastatin, Simvastatin, and Atorvastatin for Cardiovascular Disease Prevention. *American Heart Journal* 151(2): 273-281.

One Step Forward, Two Steps Back?
Taking Stock of German Health Care Reforms to Date

Biggi Bender

Abstract

German statutory health insurance is a social insurance system financed through contributions and having an influential self-administration. This results in specific problems such as deficits in the financing basis, a slow speed of innovations due to dominant corporatist structures, deep divisions between the various fields of health care, and financial risks resulting from a high concentration of doctors and hospitals. Since the 1970s, cost control has been one of the main topics of German health care policy. In contrast, the implementation of competitive elements and the support of innovations in health care supply to improve quality and efficiency have only taken place since the 1990s, but to a very limited extent and against the strong opposition from politics and the health care sector. The present federal government has close patronage relationships to groups in the health care sector who profit from the status quo. Therefore, they only show little enthusiasm for continuing the gentle process of modernisation of the last decade. On their agenda are the shift of the critical load from the employers to the employees as well as from the high earners to the low earners and thus a considerable weakening of the social character of statutory health insurance. However, this scheme is very controversially debated in German society. Concepts to link innovations on the supply side with an inclusion of all demographic groups in social insurance on the financial side meet with great approval.

Zusammenfassung

Die gesetzliche Krankenversicherung in Deutschland ist ein Sozialversicherungssystem mit Beitragsfinanzierung und ausgeprägter Selbstverwaltung. Daraus ergeben sich spezifische Probleme: Zu ihnen gehören Defizite in der Finanzierungsbasis, ein geringes Innovationstempo infolge der Dominanz korporatistischer Strukturen, tiefe Gräben zwischen den verschiedenen Versorgungsbereichen und Ausgabenrisiken, die sich aus einer überaus hohen Arzt- und Krankenhausdichte ergeben. Die Ausgabensteuerung gehört schon seit den 1970er Jahren zu den wichtigsten Themen der deutschen Gesundheitspolitik. Dagegen finden die Implementierung von Wettbewerbselementen und die Förderung von Versorgungsinnovationen zur Verbesserung der Qua-

lität und Wirtschaftlichkeit der Gesundheitsversorgung erst seit den 1990er Jahren statt – jedoch in sehr begrenztem Ausmaß und gegen erhebliche Widerstände aus der Politik und dem Gesundheitswesen. Die derzeitige Bundesregierung unterhält enge Klientelbeziehungen zu den Gruppen im Gesundheitswesen, die vom Status quo profitieren. Dementsprechend gering ist ihre Bereitschaft, den vorsichtigen Modernisierungskurs des vergangenen Jahrzehnts fortzusetzen. Auf der Agenda der Regierung steht stattdessen eine Belastungsverschiebung von den Arbeitgebern hin zu den Arbeitnehmern sowie von Gut- hin zu Geringverdienenden und damit verbunden eine deutliche Schwächung des Sozialversicherungscharakters der gesetzlichen Krankenversicherung. Allerdings ist dieses Vorhaben in der deutschen Gesellschaft sehr umstritten. Große Zustimmung finden dagegen Konzepte, die Innovationen auf der Versorgungsseite mit einer Einbeziehung aller Bevölkerungsgruppen in die Sozialversicherung auf der Finanzierungsseite verbinden.

The German health care system ranks among social insurances. The Statutory Health Insurance (SHI) is financed through income-related contributions. The government restricts itself to specifying guidelines. Detailed decisions on the catalogue of services and quality specifications are jointly made in the self-governing boards by representatives of social health insurance funds and the medical profession as well as the special interest organisation of hospitals. Services are rendered by public institutions, non-profit institutions run by charity organisations and private institutions in the hospital sector, and by mainly independent providers in the outpatient sector of which general practitioners are the most important and most influential group.

The rationale of SHI have proven successful. The SHI is comparatively independent of the federal budget due to the financing through earmarked contributions. Hence, health care is not always competing with other important political aims. The German health care system is well equipped as to material and personnel due to this type of funding. Specifying entitlements to benefits, quality standards, and remuneration structures by the representatives of third-party payers and health care providers lead to more practical relevance and acceptance from the local players than governmental top-down decisions would gain. Furthermore, the German system, relying on societal self-regulation, has lead to a broad offer of hospitals and surgeries. Waiting times for consultation or hospital treatment cannot completely be avoided but are very short as compared to many other countries.

However, a health insurance system such as the German one also shows structural risks.

- It is important to define the incomes liable to contribution in order to permanently accept and finance the system. Most systems financed by contributions will always have their constraints because of contribution ceilings for incomes. These upper income limits for contributions can be justified since a system based on income-related contributions does not have a correlation between the amount of contributions paid and the entitlement to services. This is, however, an Achilles' heel with regard to legitimising points of view. It can only be cured if the income-related principle is consequently applied to all types of income below the upper income limit for contributions. This is also important to make the financing of the system immune to changes in the income structure.

- The negotiated settlements, which are targeted in corporatist systems, are often extremely lengthy. Contradictory interests of the players involved are likely to block decisions. Subsequently, negotiation systems tend to be conservative in structure.

- Health insurer which can set the contribution level themselves and a health care system influenced by private suppliers, whose incomes largely depend on the number of invoiced services, run the risk of increasing expenses. The interest of the health care providers in their earnings is thus primarily mirrored without having a positive impact on the quality of health care.

These structural problems inherent in such a social health insurance system are to be found in the reality of SHI.

- With compulsorily insured persons in SHI, only part of the income is taken into account when calculating the contributions to health insurance. Wages and wage replacement incomes, such as pensions or unemployment benefits, are liable to contributions. However, income from capital or profit is exempt from contributions. Their share in public property has considerably grown since the 1990s. The incomes liable to contribution per member have only raised by an average of 1 per cent in SHI since 1996. In contrast, the public property – which is calculated on the basis of wages as well as incomes from companies and capital – has risen by approx. 1.8 per cent over the same period. Despite a considerable collapse (- 4.2 per cent) due to the crisis in 2009. The financial basis of SHI is breaking up like an ice floe in the sun. This is the main reason for the continuously increasing contributions in SHI. The growing demand on the health care sector due to demographic changes and medical progress has to be financed by a shrinking part of societal income.

The problem of funding is increased by the possibility of high earners, civil servants, and self-employed persons to be insured in private health insurances (PHI) and medical care of civil servants being mostly financed from tax resources. The opt-out option for high earners and the special system for civil servants result in the 10 per cent of the population having the highest incomes and the best health not participating in financing the social health insurance funds.

- The influential role of social health insurance fund associations as well as doctors' associations in organising the system has often proven to hinder innovations. Governmental decrees, such as the lump-sum-per-case system in hospitals or the introduction of the electronic health card, would have foundered on the objections of the self-governing bodies without the interference to each federal government in office. Corporatism also proves to be extremely conservative in structure with the organisation of local care. The collective agreements which have to be concluded consistently and collectively between social health insurance funds on the one hand and doctors and hospitals on the other allow only few innovations in health care. In particular, the strict separation between the inpatient and outpatient sectors, the key structural deficit of the German health care system, is continued.

- In its survey in 2000/2001, the Division Board of Experts for Concerted Action in the Public Health Sector has diagnosed health care utilisation in the German health care sector. Many patients would get too much treatment as compared to others, who would not get any at all, while yet others would be wrongly treated. According to estimates, approx. 30 per cent of all X-rays are redundant. But then again half of the patients suffering a heart attack are not treated at all. »We are paying for a Mercedes but are driving a Volkswagen Golf.« In public debate, this sentence is often quoted to describe the lack of efficiency of the German health care sector.

From the 1970s to the 1990s –
From Cost Containment to Competition between Social Health Insurance Funds

Four issues have crystallised in the German health care insurance system since the 1970s. Apart from financing, these are regulation, cost control, and efficiency with the last three topics being closely connected.

Looking at the health care reforms passed in this period, it becomes evident that cost control was an important issue in all reforms. During the 1970s and 1980s, the main focus was on achieving this aim in consent with the joint self-governing boards and other players in the health care sector, whereas governmental influence was increased in the 1990s. Remuneration in the medical outpatient sector, costs for medicinal products and remedies, and hospital remuneration were linked to the development of the incomes liable to contribution. This budgeting has ever since been part of the armoury of German health care policy in varying degrees of intensity and form. The changing federal governments have been quite successful despite public perception. The share of the gross national product in SHI expenditure has remained stable between 6 per cent and 6.5 per cent over the last 15 years.

Since the beginning of the 1990s, significant changes have also occurred with the regulation of the system. The corporate control by joint self-governing boards and state has increasingly been complemented by competitive elements. The origin of this paradigm shift was the Gesundheitsstrukturgesetz (GSG) [Health Care Structure Act] jointly passed by CDU/CSU [Christian Democratic Union of Germany/Christian Social Union of Bavaria] and SPD [Social Democratic Party of Germany] in 1992. The competition between social health insurance funds was thus introduced in the social health insurance funds. Since 1996, all statutory insured have the possibility to freely choose between all social health insurance funds.

It then became obvious that different attitudes towards competition exist in the German health care policy. The CDU/CSU wanted to stoke up competition between the social health insurance funds and encourage the insured to make economical use of the health services by offering rate options such as no-claims bonus, reimbursement of costs, or co-payment. In contrast, the SPD claimed the extension of competition by shifting from the demand side to the supply side in the health care sector. Social health insurance funds were to conclude selective contracts with individual doctors or hospitals to thus promote a so-called competition on contractual terms between the health care providers. This was considered to offer a solution to the problems of expenditure as well as efficiencies.

The Health Care Policy of SPD and Bündnis 90/Die Grünen [Alliance '90/The Greens] – Competition for Quality and Efficiency

When SPD and Bündnis 90/Die Grünen came into power in 1998, the Competition for Quality and Efficiency became government programme. Efficiency reserves in the health care sector were to be opened up mainly by more competition between the health care providers. Hospital financing was to be almost completely transferred into a lump-sum-per-case system within a few years. Thus, cost transparency was to be created and competition between hospitals encouraged. However, the intention of the SPD and Bündnis 90/Die Grünen to completely transfer medical specialists' care from a system of collective agreements into a system of selective contracting failed because of the CDU/CSU's veto, whose consent was required because they held the majority of votes in the Bundesrat [Federal Council] at that time. Nevertheless, integrated health care could be incorporated as a completely new health care sector into hospital law. Individual social health insurance funds and health care providers should thus be enabled to conclude selective contracts. The architects of the SPD and Bündnis 90/Die Grünen of the reform hoped to encourage an innovation competition.

With the health care reform in 2004, Medizinische Versorgungszentren (MVZ) [medical care units], a new type of health care facilities, were accredited. Various doctors from the same or different medical fields are working together under one roof.

The health care policy of SPD and Bündnis 90/Die Grünen was strongly oriented towards bringing about changes in the health care structures. On the one hand, this was done by direct legislative intervention, such as the reforms of remuneration structures in hospitals, the accreditation and financial promotion of co-operative health care forms, or the introduction of structured treatment programmes for chronically ill persons. On the other hand, the health care policy of SPD and Bündnis 90/Die Grünen aimed at encouraging more competition between the health care providers by creating alternatives to corporatist collective agreements. This was to serve as a so-called detection process for more quality and efficiency.

Accompanying measures were implemented to avoid unwanted consequences of competition on the system of solidarity. Hospitals and general practitioners were obliged to quality management and, additionally, hospitals also to compile quality reports. The joint self-administration got its own quality institute, the Institute for Quality and Efficiency in Health Care, and morbidity-based risk structure compensation between social health insurance funds was established.

Health Care Policy of the Great Coalition

Between 2005 and 2008, the great coalition stayed on the reform path pursued by introducing competition between social health insurance funds in the 1990s and extending it onto the supply side by the SPD and Bündnis 90/Die Grünen from 1998 onwards. This can also be attributed to the dominance of the Bundesgesundheitsministerium [Federal Ministry for Health] headed by a social-democratic minister and a CDU/CSU who had nothing comparable to counter. The health care reform of 2007 pointed at more competition because of implementing contract negotiations in the sector of therapeutic devices, the detaching of part of general practitioner care (general practitioners health care) from the collective contract system, and the extension of price negotiations between social health insurance funds and pharmaceutical companies. However, part of the union CDU/CSU was still strongly opposed to more competition between the suppliers of health care. The decision to more competition between general practitioners was undermined by de facto granting the Deutsche Hausärzteverband [German Association of General Practitioners] a contractual monopoly on the general practitioner centred care. This backward roll was initiated by the CSU – facing state elections in Bavaria and, therefore, looking for solidarity from the local Association of General Practitioners.

The great coalition had announced to solve the problem of financing SHI but failed. They only agreed on a considerable extension of governmental influence as to cost control. A global budget was de facto introduced to SHI by establishing a central health fund into which contributions to SHI are paid to be then allocated to the social insurance funds depending on the number of insured. In addition, the introduction of additional contributions opened the door for a system of lump sum per allowance per head. Though the additional contributions were restricted to 2 per cent at most of the insured's income and summed up to no more than 5 per cent of the annual expenses of the health fund, it could clearly be seen right from the start that changed majorities would enable the CDU/CSU and FDP [Free Democratic Party (Germany)] to further pave the way for a system of income-related contributions.

Health Care Reforms 1998–2008 – The Long Way to Competition

Health care policy between the government of SPD and Bündnis 90/Die Grünen starting in 1998 and the end of the great coalition and SPD in 2008 was characterised by the efforts to create more competition between the suppliers of health care as well. Besides, it was the government which tried to improve the legal and financial parameters for co-operative forms of care. However, the implementation of competitive elements into the German health care system is still at a very early stage despite the great number of reform measures. Collective contracts between social health insurance funds and the local medical profession are still predominant in the ambulatory sector, selective contracts between social health insurance funds and doctors or group practices still comprise only a very small part of health care supply. Hospitals are still governed by planned economy structures despite the lump-sum-per-case system. The introduction of competition in the field of therapeutic devices is not yet accepted, not even by the patients. Not least the social health insurance funds are to be blamed for this because they consider competition solely as an instrument for cost reduction and not as a means of innovation and quality improvement.

The slow speed of reform mainly has two reasons. First of all, the resistance of the established suppliers of health care to any change in health care structures as they recognise it as a threat to their acquired rights. The vehement protest from the medical profession against new co-operative forms of health care, for instance medical care units, which are considered to be a threat to their own existence as small business owners, has become a permanent topic in German health policy. Second, the political parties are very divided over the extent to which competition on the part of the supplier is to be expanded. CDU/CSU and FDP have close patronage relationships to that part of the medical profession who profit from the status quo.

The interest of the Bundesländer [Laender] adds to this. They do not want to ease their grip on the hospital sector. Therefore, they persistently reject the implementation of selective contracts between social health insurance funds and hospitals.

Against this backdrop, it cannot finally be evaluated whether and to which extent the reform measures with regard to competition and supply policy have contributed to improve cost control and efficiency in the German health care sector since 1998. It is, however, a fact that increased competition in the pharmaceutical sector, or rather the generic segment, has led to major price cuts. But these were overcompensated by exorbitant price increases with brand name drugs. Since the price negotiations only started at the beginning of the year, their impact in this pharmaceutical sector remains to be seen. The introduction of disease management programmes seems to have led to an improvement in the care of severely ill patients and thus also given a positive impetus for the treatment of chronically ill patients not taking part in these programmes. The excessive lengths of stay in German hospitals have also been reduced. The effects of more competition and co-operation on the German health system can only be reliably evaluated in a few years' time. This is a major task for health care research as well.

The by far largest area requiring improvement in German health care policy is the financing of SHI. No federal government has yet had the courage to tackle this reform task due to its large potential for conflict. Instead, health policy became some kind of patchwork: one so-called patch was the co-payment as independent financial backbone implemented in the 1980s. Another was a tax-financed federal grant to SHI, implemented by the SPD and Bündnis 90/Die Grünen in 2004. Both have their limits. Co-payment is in a conflicting relationship to the principle of solidarity between the healthy and the sick as well as the high earners and the low earners. The expansion of complementary tax-financing is not a realistic option in view of the record deficit in the public purse. Apart from that, SHI would then become dependent on the federal budget.

Two Steps Back – The Health Care Reform of 2010

Last year's health care reform adopted by CDU/CSU [Christian Democratic Union of Germany/Christian Social Union of Bavaria] and FDP [Free Democratic Party (Germany)] constitutes a break. The surcharges, implemented by the previous government, became the starting point for a comprehensive change of the system under the coalition. The income-related contribution rate was frozen. Increase in expenses will in future be solely financed through flat-rate surcharges. These are exclusively paid by the insured without any participation of the employer. The social equity among the health insured for the sector of surcharges is to be separated from SHI and, in the medium term, financed through the fiscal system. The financing of SHI will thus gradually be converted from income-related contributions to flat-rate premiums. The principle of parity, i.e. the financing of the contributions on a fifty-fifty basis between insured and employers, will become obsolescent. The coalition partners will adhere to the separation of SHI and private health insurances. The change to private health insurance will become easier for high-income employees.

This subtle system change will have a significant effect on the distribution policy. In the short and medium terms, high-income earners will have to pay less whereas low-income earners will have to pay more due to the system of flat-rate premiums. In the long term, the continuously decreasing financial share of the employers will lead to increasing contributions also for high-income earners. Most notably, by detaching social equity, SHI will increasingly lose their character of a social insurance. According to the wording of the law adopted, the insured are to get social equity if the average surcharges exceeds 2 per cent of the income liable to contribution. In future, the federal budget will have to increasingly finance SHI. Today, the tax component of SHI amounts to approx. 8 per cent. This share would reach the 20 per cent limit within the next ten years with a social equity conceived by the federal government. This would, of course, have an impact on the control of SHI. It would move towards a state-controlled system.

However, the reform shows all the features of a mere formulaic compromise between the coalition parties. Even the proponents of this reform do not know how to reliably finance the social equity through the federal budget. In view of the record deficit of the federal government, permanent arguments on the conditions of entitlement and the level of social equity are inevitable. The heated debate on the future financing of SHI has not yet been finished despite the passing of the reform.

The health reform 2010 does not give any answers to the control and efficiency problems of SHI. The federal government announced to catch up on these reforms in a so-called care supply act in the course of this year. In the meantime, there is a key issue paper for this parliamentary bill of the Federal Ministry for Health. The term competition is solely used in connection with the social health insurance funds. In future, these are to be entitled to offer additional services beyond the catalogue of services. More competition between the suppliers of health care is, however, not envisaged in the ministry's reform plan. This is evidence of a halved understanding of competition which has been characteristic of the health policy by the CDU/CSU coalition of the 1990s. This way to understand the health care sector seems to still have a guiding effect, at least in the FDP, who has a close patronage relationship with medical specialists.

Solidarity and Competition – The Reform Alternative

In view of a demographic change and the progress in medical technology, the access of everyone to medically necessary health care supply can only be guaranteed if the system becomes much more efficient. These improvements in efficiency will only be achieved if the control structures are altered. Special significance must be attached to the extension of competitive elements. It will also be important that state and legislature offer additional incentives for innovations in health care. This comprises the adjustment of remuneration structures in the different fields of the health care sector or the expansion of health care research. But this also means that social health insurance funds will get the financial scope to invest in the innovations of health care. A global budget preset by the government, as introduced by the great coalition [CDU/CSU and SPD] with the health fund and the uniform contribution rate, will be obstructive. It has already become apparent that the social health insurance funds do everything to manage as long as possible with the allocations of the health fund. Otherwise, they are forced to charge high surcharges so that they will drop behind in the competition between the social health care funds. It will thus hardly be possible to mobilise funds for the set-up of new supply structures.

Competition does not necessarily lower expenses. Competition may lead to more efficiency and a faster pace of innovation with suitable parameters. Intelligent cost control will in future also be required in SHI.

Furthermore, a financial reform is required to cope with the deficiencies of the German SHI without jeopardising their strength. This includes the basis for contribution assessment on all kinds of income, the inclusion of all demographic groups in social equity, and the generation of a uniform market of social health insurance funds (Bürgerversicherung [citizens' insurance]). Such a reform is necessary for both a lasting acceptance and the possibility of financing SHI.

The discussion on the reform perspectives will continue to determine health policy in Germany over the next few years.

World Champion in Health Care Reforms – Impact of German Health Care Policy on the Statutory Health Insurance

Norbert Klusen

Abstract

Germany is world champion in reforming the health care system. On the one hand, these reforms are necessary to break up encrusted and outmoded structures within the system and to make room for new intelligent solutions. In recent years German health policy has been successful in controlling costs and has introduced more competition and contractual freedom in health care. On the other hand, too many single acts, too much regulation and a too finely spun web of central control hinder the necessary innovation and readiness for change of all stakeholders. Therefore, health policy needs greater confidence in the positive power of competition instead of focusing on detailed short-term legal intervention. Quality transparency, new competitive tools and increasing orientation towards scientific information are key success factors that will influence the sustainable development of the German health care system in the future.

Zusammenfassung

Deutschland ist Weltmeister im Bereich Gesundheitsreformen. Einerseits sind diese Reformen notwendig, um die verkrusteten und veralteten Strukturen innerhalb des Systems aufzubrechen und Raum für neue, intelligente Lösungen zu schaffen. Die Kostendämpfungsmaßnahmen der letzten Jahre haben geholfen, die Beitragssätze und damit die Lohnnebenkosten zu stabilisieren. Zusätzlich wurde ab 1996 der Grundstein für mehr Wettbewerb und Vertragsfreiheit im deutschen Gesundheitswesen gelegt. Andererseits behindern zu viele einzelne Gesetze, zu viel Regulierung und ein zu fein gesponnenes Netz zentralistischer Kontrolle die Innovationsfähigkeit und Veränderungsbereitschaft aller Akteure. Deshalb braucht die Gesundheitspolitik mehr Vertrauen in die positive Kraft des Wettbewerbs, statt sich auf kurzfristige gesetzliche Regulierungen zu konzentrieren. Qualitätstransparenz, neue Wettbewerbsinstrumente und eine wachsende Ausrichtung auf wissenschaftliche Informationen sind Schlüsselfaktoren, die die Entwicklung des deutschen Gesundheitssystems in Zukunft nachhaltig beeinflussen werden.

Germany is a world champion in the field of health care reforms. In contrast to other countries, the German state regularly intervenes, at increasingly frequent intervals, in the financial and organisational structures of health insurance and long-term care insurance, both statutory. Indeed, over the past four years alone, a total of eleven major reforms and legislative initiatives have fundamentally changed the health care system. Alongside Pflegeweiterentwicklungsreform [Reform of the Advancement of Long-term Care Insurance] and Krankenhausfinanzierungsreform [Reform of Hospital Financing], the reorganisation of insolvency law for social health insurance funds, and the 15th amendment to the Medical Preparations Act, it is largely the GKV-Wettbewerbsstärkungsgesetz (GKV-WSG) [Statutory Health Insurance Competition Strengthening Act] and, following the change of coalition, the Gesetz zur Neuordnung des Arzneimittelmarktes (AMNOG) [Act for the Restructuring of the Pharmaceutical Market] and the GKV-Finanzierungsgesetz (GKV-FinG) [Statutory Health Insurance Financing Act] that have shaped the debate on the sustainable development of the German health care sector.

The catalogue of benefits has also been repeatedly supplemented with important measures, such as preventive check-ups or, as part of the fifth branch of the social insurance scheme, personal long-term care insurance. However, the main focus of political efforts in health care since the 1980s, regardless of the political party, has been on stabilising the contribution rates and so-called ancillary wage costs through cost-containment measures.

Hence in 1983, millions of pensioners, who had so far complementarily been insured, were required to pay contributions through the German Pension Adjustment Act. Benefit cuts for dental prostheses, spectacles, medicinal products, and death benefit were made, and out-of-pocket payments, particularly for medication and hospital treatment, were introduced. Savings were also made on doctors, the pharmaceutical industry, and clinics, a hospital emergency contribution of 20 DM was introduced and the so-called Praxisgebühr [a practice fee for visits to the doctor] was implemented in 2004.

Already in 2005, the former German Federal Minister of Health, Ulla Schmidt, heralded the end of financing on equal terms with the introduction of a special contribution of 0.9 per cent solely for insured. In 2009, this was cemented through the establishment of additional contributions, and in 2010, by freezing the employers' contributions.

In addition to cost-containment policies, 1996 fortunately also saw the foundation being laid for increased competition within the health care sector. It was made obligatory for social health insurance funds to accept almost all applicants. In the meantime, social health insurance funds are allowed to merge with social health insurance funds from other associations. The resulting competitive pressure caused a marked reduction in the number of social health insurance funds. In 1990, there were more than 1,000 active funds, and with just 160 today, an end to this concentration process is not yet in sight.

As a result of this development, customer needs, service management, and administrative efficiency have, for many years, been among the everyday concerns of German social health insurance funds.

In addition to competition among social health insurance funds, the way has also slowly but steadily been paved for more freedom of contract within the statutory health insurance system. Alongside rebate contracts, which have recently been adopted under German antitrust law, the insured have the option of voluntarily entering into integrated health care contracts and negotiating individually tailored optional tariffs. In contrast, the straitjacket of obligatory primary physician contracts and the Disease Management Programme (DMP), as instruments of financial equalisation, have nothing to do with competition and, up to now, have failed to achieve an improvement in health care structures. In the main, the new competitive instruments also remain restricted to outpatient services and medicinal products. As the biggest cost driver in the health care system, hospital services continue to be excluded.

On the one hand, the upshot of this kaleidoscope of reform efforts is that Germany is by far the most successful of the OECD member countries in terms of cost containment, a fact that has benefitted the insured and employers. The costs of statutory health insurance, based on the level of the gross domestic product, have remained stable for many years.

There is also evidence that the competitive options first introduced into the German health care system have led to positive restlessness and clear structural improvements. Social health insurance funds evaluate their position on the market and thus they encourage one another to improve. Rebate contracts for medicinal products have already resulted in savings worth hundreds of millions of Euros, while integrated health care contracts have led to quality competition and a greater focus on innovation. The choice of optional tariffs and hence a marked difference in the range of services help to keep those insured, whose income is above the compulsory insurance income threshold, to remain within the solidarity system of statutory health insurance.

Thus the health care reforms and laws have not principally been amiss. On the other hand, the increasing speed of the reform process and the non-uniform health care politics of different parties and party groups also clearly demonstrate the following:

• Financial pressure is still present within the system and it will be difficult to control it through pure cost containment. There is growing realisation that comprehensive health care for all is unlikely to become any cheaper in the future.

- To date, a shared, long-term cross-party vision for the future development of the statutory health insurance is still lacking in Germany. The decision as to whether more state regulation or rather more competition can turn health care into a self-regulating, learning system, does not appear to have been concluded as yet. As such, the equalising distribution mechanisms of a health fund and the morbidity-based risk structure compensation are in diametric opposition to the new competitive options. Similarly, the centralistic formation of a Spitzenverband Bund [Federal Association of Statutory Health Insurance Funds] is in opposition to the act of opening social health insurance funds, and the lack of a uniformly operating supervisory authority to ensure the same competitive conditions throughout Germany is in opposition to selective contract options.
- For this reason, the reliability of the health policy is only available in part. Providing the decisions to further develop German statutory health insurance are made on the basis of political expediencies rather than scientific findings, in other words, as long as ideologies have priority over the consideration of objective facts, social health insurance funds have to expect the wheel of the system to take a sudden turn in a completely different direction in the event of a change of government. This makes the ability to plan corporate decisions unnecessarily difficult within statutory health insurance.

A look beyond Germany shows that other countries are quicker to achieve the goals set to reform their health care systems.

The Netherlands boasts a long-term, cross-party vision of a generally and competitively oriented health care system. In 2006, the insured were afforded a strong market position. Under the scrutiny of a uniform regulatory body, the health insurance funds are currently permitted to try out completely different competitive instruments for all health care sectors. This makes the strengths and weaknesses of this range of services more transparent, while the insights gained from this transparency help to continually develop the system.

Quality improvement is a key topic in England. The quality of medical care is monitored over the long term and consequences can be expected if quality standards fail to be adhered to. As the current White Paper by the Secretary of State for Health, Andrew Lansley, demonstrates, the coalition government is now involved in revitalising its internal market by introducing *general practice commissioning consortia*.

In Germany, many parties still hugely underestimate the opportunities and positive pressure of competition from a political point of view. Alongside the funding reform, it would therefore be wise to consider the structural reform of the system in terms of the following questions:

- How is it possible to create more transparency concerning the quality of medical care financed by the German statutory health insurance system? Only by knowing the quality of health services available can these be improved and good quality rewarded accordingly. Hence, the demand for more quality transparency in the »black box« of outpatient services is not an end in itself, but ultimately a matter of patient protection. For this reason, quality needs to be measurable and must become a key topic of the future.
- In the future, which new competitive instruments will be available to previously excluded health care sectors, in order to stimulate the system's innovation focus and its willingness to adapt change?
- How do we overcome the resisting power of the political system towards the rational basis of scientific information gained from studies and evaluations, so that Germany does not remain an importing country for this kind of knowledge?

There will always be health care reforms. They are important for breaking set and outdated structures in the system and for creating space for intelligent, new solutions. Too many individual laws, too much regulation and overly complicated centralised control certainly harm the need for innovation and the willingness to adapt change among all players within the health care system.

The future organisation of German statutory health insurance remains an important reform topic and a key topic for the next federal election campaign.

We should confidentially offer our title as world champions in the field of health care reforms and focus instead on achieving a new balance: Between a state that restricts itself to the parameters of the legal and institutional framework and the compliance with its rules and refrains from detailed short-term intervention, and the opportunities and strength of a self-regulating, learning system in competition.

Chapter 2:
Competition or Collaboration –
Benefits for English and German Patients?

Health Care reform in the UK's National Health Service

Jennifer Dixon, Judith Smith, Anita Charlesworth, Martin Bardsley

Abstract

The recent White Paper Equity and Excellence: Liberating the NHS (Department of Health, 2010) sets out the next reform programme for the NHS in England. The resulting Health Bill is currently progressing through parliament. The reforms will be implemented in a period of significant financial challenge for the NHS. As set out in the recent Spending Review (HM Treasury, 2010) the NHS will receive 0.4 per cent real terms growth over the next four years to 2014/5 – i.e. 0.1 per cent per year. This compares to an average real terms increase of 5.7 per cent from 1997/8 to 2009/10. This is the lowest four years' increase for the NHS since 1951–1956 (Emmerson et al., 2010). The Spending Review allocates £ 1 billion a year from NHS funding to social care. The real terms change in the NHS funding net of the social care support is a reduction of 0.5 per cent over the next four years.

The main goals in the White Paper and the Spending Review are: to uphold the values and principles of the NHS (of a comprehensive service, available to all, free at the point of use and based on clinical need and not on the ability to pay); to increase health spending in real terms in each year of this parliament; and for the NHS to achieve results that are amongst the best in the world.

The NHS embarks on this period of financial challenge and reform with many strengths. Research by the Commonwealth Fund (Commonwealth Fund, 2009) comparing six countries shows that the UK has moved from third position to first across a range of attributes including quality of care, efficiency and equity. The NHS has never been better resourced, waiting times have fallen dramatically and public satisfaction with the service is high (NatCen, 2009). But whilst funding has risen considerably over the last decade, by international standards, the NHS does not look lavishly funded. At the start of the banking crisis spending on health as a share of GDP had grown from 6.6 per cent in 1996 to 8.7 per cent in 2008, to just below the Organisation for Economic Co-operation and Development (OECD) average and lower than many other major economies (OECD, 2009). In terms of real resources the NHS still has fewer doctors, hospital beds and key equipment such as MRI and CT scanners per head of population than the OECD average. But while resources matter, the service should be judged on outcomes not inputs. Life expectancy has been improving in the UK, life expectancy at birth in England and Wales has increased over the last two decades by 5.3 years for men and 3.8 years for women. Despite this the UK has a relatively high rate of mortality amenable to health care and compares less favourably with other OECD countries on measures of health status and in critical areas such as cancer survival rates (Anderson and Maskovich, 2010; Leatherman and Sutherland, 2008).

Over the next four years the pressures on the NHS will continue to rise. Previous work (Appleby et al., 2009; Wanless, 2002) on financial pressures has identified the following key factors:

* demography – England has a growing and ageing population;
* pay and price pressures;
* new technologies;
* rising expectations and quality.

Meeting these challenges so that the NHS can sustain the access to services and quality of care will require the NHS to make substantial efficiency and productivity gains. The Spending Review increases for the NHS are consistent with the requirement for the NHS to make efficiency savings of £ 15-20 billion over the next four years (Nicholson, 2009). This is equivalent to around 4 and 5 per cent year. The Government's proposed reforms to the NHS will be a success if they help the NHS to live within the tighter resources while continuing to improve quality and health outcomes.

Zusammenfassung

Das letzte Weißbuch Equity and Excellence: Liberating the NHS [Eigenkapital und Güte: Liberalisierung des britischen Gesundheitswesens] (Department of Health, 2010) beschreibt das nächste Reformprogramm des NHS in England. Die daraus resultierende Gesetzesvorlage wird gerade im Parlament beraten. Die Reformen werden in einer Zeit bedeutender finanzieller Herausforderungen für den NHS umgesetzt werden. Wie im letzten Spending Review [Haushaltsplan] (HM Treasury, 2010) dargelegt, wird der NHS um real 0,4 Prozent über die nächsten vier Jahre, bis 2014/15, wachsen, d. h. um 0,1 Prozent pro Jahr. Das entspricht einem realen Wachstum von 5,7 Prozent zwischen 1997/98 und 2009/10. Das ist das niedrigste Wachstum des NHS innerhalb von vier Jahren seit dem Spending Review 1951–1956 (Emmerson et al., 2010). Der Spending Review weist von den Geldern des NHS jährlich £ 1 Milliarde der Sozialfürsorge zu. Real bedeutet diese Änderung bei der finanziellen Zuweisung für den NHS zur Unterstützung der Sozialfürsorge netto eine Reduktion von 0,5 Prozent über die nächsten vier Jahre.

Die Hauptziele im Weißbuch und im Spending Review sind, die Werte und Grundsätze des NHS aufrechtzuerhalten (ein umfassender Service für alle, kostenfrei und basierend auf dem klinischen Bedarf und nicht auf der Zahlungsfähigkeit); ein reales Wachstum der Zuweisungen an den NHS in jedem Jahr dieser Regierung sowie Ergebnisse zu erreichen, die zu den besten der Welt zählen.

In dieser Zeit der finanziellen Herausforderungen und Reformen zeigt der NHS viele Stärken. Der Commonwealth Fund [eine private Stiftung für ein hochqualifiziertes Gesundheitssystem] (Commenwealth Fund, 2009) hat sechs Länder verglichen und dabei festgestellt, dass Großbritannien auf den Gebieten der Pflegequalität, der Effizienz und des Eigenkapitals vom dritten auf den ersten Platz vorgerückt ist. Der NHS war nie besser aufgestellt, die Wartezeiten sind dramatisch gesunken und die Zufriedenheit der Bevölkerung mit dem Service ist hoch (NatCen, 2009). Obwohl die finanziellen Ressourcen im internationalen Vergleich während der letzten zehn Jahre beträchtlich gestiegen sind, verfügt der NHS nicht über großzügige Mittel. Zu Beginn der Finanzkrise waren die Gesundheitsausgaben als Teil des Bruttosozialproduktes von 6,6 Prozent 1996 auf 8,7 Prozent 2008 gestiegen, ein Wert kurz unter dem des von der Organisation für wirtschaftliche Zusammenarbeit und Entwicklung (OECD) angegebenen Durchschnittswerts und niedriger als in vielen anderen bedeutenden Wirtschaftsnationen (OECD, 2009). Hinsichtlich der realen Ressourcen hat der NHS immer noch weniger Ärzte sowie weniger Krankenhausbetten und ist schlechter ausgestattet mit wichtigen Geräten wie MRT und CT pro Kopf der Bevölkerung als der OECD-Durchschnitt. Auch wenn die Ressourcen wichtig sind, so sollte der Service nach Ergebnis und nicht nach Eingabe bewertet werden. Die Lebenserwartung ist in Großbritannien gestiegen, die Lebenserwartung bei der Geburt ist in den letzten beiden Jahrzehnten in England und Wales um 5,3 Jahre bei Männern und um 3,8 Jahre bei Frauen gestiegen. Trotzdem hat Großbritannien eine hohe Rate vermeidbarer Sterbefälle in der medizinischen Versorgung und schneidet im Vergleich mit anderen OECD-Ländern bei Indikatoren zum Gesundheitsstatus sowie in kritischen Bereichen, wie bspw. der Überlebensrate bei Krebs, wenig vorteilhaft ab (Anderson und Maskovich, 2010; Leatherman und Sutherland, 2008).

Innerhalb der nächsten vier Jahre wird der Druck auf den NHS weiter steigen. In bisherigen Veröffentlichungen zum finanziellen Druck (Appleby et al., 2009; Wanless, 2002) wurden folgende Schlüsselfaktoren ermittelt:

- Demografie – England hat eine wachsende und alternde Bevölkerung
- Vergütungs- und Preisdruck
- neue Technologien
- steigende Erwartungen und Qualität

Um sich diesen Herausforderungen zu stellen, so dass der NHS den Zugang zu Service und Pflegequalität aufrechterhalten kann, wird er substantielle Gewinne bei Effizienz und Produktivität machen müssen. Die Erhöhungen im Spending Review für den NHS stimmen mit den Forderungen an den NHS überein, Einsparungen von £ 15 bis 20 Milliarden über die nächsten vier Jahre zu machen (Nicholson, 2009). Das entspricht etwa 4–5 Prozent pro Jahr. Die Reformvorschläge der Regierung für den NHS werden erfolgreich sein, wenn sie dem NHS helfen, mit begrenzteren Mitteln zu leben und gleichzeitig die Qualität und Gesundheitsversorgung zu verbessern.

Background basic information

The UK's National Health Service (NHS) covers England, Scotland, Wales and Northern Ireland. The policy of devolution in 1997 means that the approach to reform of the NHS in each country is now different across each country. Also since 1997 there has been significant investment in the NHS, amounting to on average 5.5 per cent real terms growth each year (compared to a long run 3 per cent real terms increase since 1948). Since 1991 more market-oriented reforms were introduced in the NHS, which after 1997 were reversed in Wales, Scotland and Northern Ireland, and were developed further in England. The remainder of this paper refers to reforms in the NHS in England.

The NHS is funded almost totally by central taxation and national insurance receipts. In 2010 the budget was £ 107 billion, and of that only about £ 500m is raised through co-payments (largely through prescription charges). All individuals in England eligible for NHS cover (all residents legally entitled to reside in England) are registered with a general practice (there are 8,100 in England). There are approximately 200 acute hospitals, and half of these are 'Foundation Trusts', which have extra freedoms over other NHS Trusts, for example to run their affairs more independently from the NHS.

NHS health care (primary, secondary and community) is commissioned by Primary Care Trusts (PCTs), of which there are 150 in England covering approximately 300,000 population. PCTs are arranged geographically – patients have no choice of PCT commissioner but are just assigned on the basis of residence. In the administrative hierarchy, above the PCTs there are ten strategic health authorities (SHAs), to which PCTs are accountable. The SHAs are accountable directly to the Department of Health.

Performance is 'managed' in England through a hierarchical relationship between the Department of Health, the SHAs and the PCTs. General practices are private businesses, but most are under an exclusive contract with the NHS which is managed by the local PCT. NHS Trusts are accountable to the PCT commissioner for performance against contract, but for financial and other matters (e.g. for hospital-acquired infection rates) are accountable to the local SHA. NHS Foundation Trusts are accountable to a Foundation Trust regulator, Monitor, for financial performance and quality of care provided. A national quality regulator, the Care Quality Commission assesses the quality of care provided in all NHS and Foundation Trusts, and publishes regular information on this.

The main pattern of reform across England since 2000 has been to encourage greater competition between hospitals in a fixed-price market, and encourage greater patient choice. There has been increased encouragement of non-NHS providers to enter the 'NHS market', with some success particularly in providing elective care. Yet still at most only 1 per cent of NHS funds are spent on non-NHS providers.

A new government was elected in May 2010, which is a coalition between the Conservative and Liberal Democrat parties. Their plans for reforming the NHS were set out in a White Paper *Equity and Excellence: Liberating the NHS* (Department of Health, 2010) which is the subject of this paper. There are four main elements of the White Paper and subsequent Bill: new arrangements for commissioning involving handing almost all commissioning to groups of general practices (GP Consortia) accountable to a new NHS Commissioning Board; encouraging all hospitals to become foundation Trusts and encouraging more competition between them (including price competition); changing the arrangements by which health care can be locally accountable; and setting up a national framework of outcomes indicators. The Bill is controversial because it represents massive upheaval in the NHS at a time of economic challenge.

Introduction

The recent White Paper *Equity and Excellence: Liberating the NHS* (Department of Health, 2010) sets out the next reform programme for the NHS in England. The resulting Health Bill is currently progressing through parliament. The reforms will be implemented in a period of significant financial challenge for the NHS. As set out in the recent *Spending Review* (HM Treasury, 2010) the NHS will receive 0.4 per cent real terms growth over the next four years to 2014/5 – i.e. 0.1 per cent per year. This compares to an average real terms increase of 5.7 per cent from 1997/8 to 2009/10. This is the lowest four years' increase for the NHS since 1951–1956 (Emmerson et al., 2010). The Spending Review allocates £ 1 billion a year from NHS funding to social care. The real terms change in the NHS funding net of the social care support is a *reduction* of 0.5 per cent over the next four years.

The main goals in the White Paper and the Spending Review are: to uphold the values and principles of the NHS (of a comprehensive service, available to all, free at the point of use and based on clinical need and not on the ability to pay); to increase health spending in real terms in each year of this parliament; and for the NHS to achieve results that are amongst the best in the world.

The NHS embarks on this period of financial challenge and reform with many strengths. Research by the Commonwealth Fund (Commonwealth Fund, 2009) comparing six countries shows that the UK has moved from third position to first across a range of attributes including quality of care, efficiency and equity. The NHS has never been better resourced, waiting times have fallen dramatically and public satisfaction with the service is high (NatCen, 2009). But whilst funding has risen considerably over the last decade, by international standards, the NHS does not look lavishly funded. At the start of the banking crisis spending on health as a share of GDP had grown from 6.6 per cent in 1996 to 8.7 per cent in 2008, to just below the Organisation for Economic Co-operation and Development (OECD) average and lower than many other major economies (OECD, 2009). In terms of real resources the NHS still has fewer doctors, hospital beds and key equipment such as MRI and CT scanners per head of population than the OECD average. But while resources matter, the service should be judged on outcomes not inputs. Life expectancy has been improving in the UK, life expectancy at birth in England and Wales has increased over the last two decades by 5.3 years for men and 3.8 years for women. Despite this the UK has a relatively high rate of mortality amenable to health care and compares less favourably with other OECD countries on measures of health status and in critical areas such as cancer survival rates (Anderson and Maskovich, 2010; Leatherman and Sutherland, 2008).

Over the next four years the pressures on the NHS will continue to rise. Previous work (Appleby et al., 2009; Wanless, 2002) on financial pressures has identified the following key factors:

• demography – England has a growing and ageing population;
• pay and price pressures;
• new technologies;
• rising expectations and quality.

Meeting these challenges so that the NHS can sustain the access to services and quality of care will require the NHS to make substantial efficiency and productivity gains. The Spending Review increases for the NHS are consistent with the requirement for the NHS to make efficiency savings of £ 15-20 billion over the next four years (Nicholson, 2009). This is equivalent to around 4 and 5 per cent year. The Government's proposed reforms to the NHS will be a success if they help the NHS to live within the tighter resources while continuing to improve quality and health outcomes.

This brief paper examines the main two elements to the government's reform programme, and then assesses whether these reforms are likely to achieve the efficiency savings now urgently needed.

Main elements of the White Paper equity and Excellence: Liberating the NHS

The White Paper emphasises GP commissioning and enhanced competition/ choice as the main reforms to improve quality and efficiency in the NHS.

(i)   GP commissioning
GP Commissioning Consortia
Across England currently care is 'commissioned' by 150 PCTs. These bodies are responsible for contracting with providers for care on behalf of the population residing within their geographical boundaries (approximately 300,000). They do so using tax funds raised centrally through general taxation and national insurance contributions, and there is no local power to raise further funds through taxation or co-payments. Individuals currently do not have a choice of NHS PCT commissioner, but are assigned a commissioner on the basis of where they live. PCTs are accountable for funds spent and performance to a higher level administrative body, a strategic health authority, which in turn is accountable to the Department of Health.

Under the current reform proposals, strategic health authorities will be abolished from 2012, and PCTs will be abolished from 2013. Instead between £ 70-80 bn of NHS funds for commissioning will be managed by 'GP Commissioning Consortia' – conglomerates of general practices. All practices are mandated to join a consortium (only one) but can choose which one they join. There is no required size of Consortia, although to date about 700 have formed with an average population covered of about 80,000. They will be accountable nationally to a new NHS Commissioning Board, which will also commission high-cost specialised services, as well as have several other functions such as resource allocation to GP Consortia, defining a failure regime for Consortia, managing primary care contracts and arranging appropriate risk sharing arrangements.

There is now nearly 20 years of evidence on the impact of primary care-led commissioning in the NHS. It points to the significant potential of GP commissioning consortia holding real, as opposed to indicative, capitated budgets for the purchasing of some local health services (and in particular community and intermediate care), and for these groups to be held to account for health outcomes, patient experience of services, and financial performance (Smith et al., 2010). It also shows that while there has been some success in improving out-of-hospital care (and electives in terms at least of more controlled referrals), commissioners have been unable to have much influence on urgent care or overall hospital efficiency. Most NHS expenditure occurs in hospitals where much greater efficiencies are urgently needed. Evidence from less radical but similar policies in the past – GP fundholding, total purchasing, primary care groups, practice-based commissioning – also shows that such approaches take time to develop and significant management and analytical resource is needed to support them (Smith et al., 2010; House of Commons, 2010; Smith et al., 2004). GP consortia will need to develop and move on significantly from their predecessors if they are to be more successful in this respect (Audit Commission, 2009).

PCTs have struggled to control expenditure on hospital care (Audit Commission, 2009). GP consortia in their early years will be underdeveloped as commissioners, handling about £ 70 bn of public funds, and subject to greater financial pressure as PCTs but with much less management resource.

There is a consensus across the developed world that key pressures on demand for health care in future will come from increasing numbers of frail older people in the population, and those with long-term conditions (Sassi and Hurst, 2008). In these population groups there are large numbers of preventable hospitalisations. It has also long been recognised that the way that health systems are organised and financed also has significant impact on expenditure. To achieve better quality and value in health care now and in the future, health systems must be incentivised towards supporting people at home so that costly avoidable hospitalisation is reduced.

As recent reviews of commissioning have shown (Audit Commission and Healthcare Commission, 2008; Smith et al., 2010; House of Commons, 2010), commissioning in the NHS has largely failed to achieve this goal, mostly because of a lack of influence over the activities of hospitals in which most expenditure occurs. Over one-third of all admissions to hospitals are emergencies accounting for some 10 per cent of NHS spending (Blunt et al., 2010). Nuffield Trust analysis shows these have risen by 11.8 per cent over five years – faster than the rise in illness levels – mainly due to very short stay admissions (Blunt et al., 2010). Commissioning has largely failed to stem this rise.

To have more effect on expenditure and quality, GPs will need to work together with specialists, patients, and indeed local authority social services to reorientate care. This is a mixture of commissioning and provision. GPs who commission are likely to need to expand their own and other community services and work with hospital clinicians in the provision of care (Smith et al., 2009; Lewis et al., 2010). Care needs to be integrated and coordinated along a pathway stretching from home to hospital, with an appropriate degree of patient choice. The Commonwealth Fund's Commission on a High Performing Health System consistently points to integrated care being the route to better value care (Commission for High Performance Health System, 2006), something underlined by Dr Denis Cortese, the outgoing chief executive of the Mayo Clinic, a health system based in the US known globally for providing first class care (Cortese, 2010), and Dr Glen Steele, CEO of another well recognised high-performing health organisation – Geisinger Health System (Steele, 2010). Key ingredients of high-performing health systems include good leadership, clinical leadership and peer review, aligned incentives, good use of information technologies for both continuous improvement work and external accountability (Baker et al., 2008). A key test of the new reform programme is the extent to which it will allow needed integration of care.

NHS Commissioning Board (NHSCB)

The NHSCB will have a critical role as the overall funder of NHS commissioners, undertaking resource allocation, designing evidence-based templates for services, and holding GP commissioners to account for their performance against the NHS Outcomes Framework (a new set of national 'outcome indicators' assessing the quality of care). It is as yet unclear how the role of the Board will relate to the economic regulator (see below section on competition) and the national body assessing the quality of care in institutions (the Care Quality Commission), and roles and principles of engagement still need to be worked out carefully. The White Paper is clear that the NHSCB will not be the 'headquarters' of the NHS, but its relationship and control over GP consortia will be critical, particularly in a tense financial climate. If a consortium or group of consortia are unable to contain expenditure or manage difficult decisions locally for example on service configurations, the Board will need to intervene, although such intervention may well demotivate the consortia, and reduce clinical engagement.

Thus a key challenge within the new arrangements is how hard choices will be made, and who will be held responsible for these. Several key issues include the following. First, whether the NHSCB will be able to remain truly independent of the Secretary of State and the Department of Health when faced with difficult local rationing decisions. Second, whether the powers of direction the NHSCB has over GP consortia will be formally set out and limited. Third, the extent to which there should be public representation on the Board of the NHSCB and/or public involvement in its decisions should also be made explicit.

The NHSCB will need to develop a failure regime for GP Consortia. The NHSCB will hold the individual general practice contracts for GPs as providers, as well as holding GP consortia to account. This poses a question as to whether and how these two areas of general practice activity will be jointly overseen at national level, and in turn how effective integration of primary care commissioning and provision can be assured.

(ii)   Competition between providers

The White Paper and subsequent Health and Social Care Bill is very strong on encouraging greater competition between hospitals. At present approximately half of all acute hospitals are foundation trusts – that is, their assets are owned by the NHS, but the management have significant independence in the way they work compared to other hospitals. For example foundation trust hospitals are not 'performance managed' by the local strategic health authority. The White Paper makes clear that the intention is for all hospitals to have foundation status by 2014.

The White Paper also makes clear that the current national body which regulates foundation trusts (this body is called Monitor) should turn into a more fully fledged economic regulator with main roles to set prices, promote competition where appropriate and ensure continuity of essential 'designated' services (these are to be defined locally). On prices, the NHS in England sets fixed prices (a national tariff) for most hospital clinical services, but the White Paper also makes clear that the regulator can in future set maximum prices, in effect allowing price competition.

There is emerging evidence that competition between hospitals, in a *fixed* price market (not using *maximum* prices), is associated with increases in quality (Gaynor, 2006; Cooper et al., 2010; Gaynor et al., 2010; Bloom et al., 2010). There is also evidence that price competition results in a decrease in quality of care, because quality is less observable than price and cost. So the move to allow maximum prices is worrying.

Similarly the new economic regulator will need to think carefully about the optimal unit of competition. Although individual hospitals are an obvious entity for competition purposes, as reflected in the White Paper, they have many different 'product lines'. The evidence for the effectiveness of competition is mostly drawn from cases where there has been increased competition for specific services, such as elective care (Gaynor, 2006; Cooper et al., 2010; Gaynor et al., 2010), including introducing new 'niche' players, rather than from a single institution.

Moreover, perhaps the biggest challenge now and into the future is caring for older people and for people with long-term conditions. As the DH, Royal Colleges and others recognise (Department of Health, 2005; Royal College of Physicians (RCP) et al., 2004; RCP, 2008), GPs need to work together with specialists so that costly avoidable hospitalisation is reduced and care is integrated and coordinated along a pathway stretching from home to hospital. Although this has been recognised across Europe and the US, countries are challenged to achieve better value from health care expenditures through better coordination and, in some cases, integrated provider networks (Stremikis et al., 2010).

The economic regulator will need to consider how it can use its powers and what the unit of competition should be to achieve improvements in unplanned care and for those with long-term conditions as well as elective and community services, drawing on international evidence. Competition between integrated providers or services may produce better efficiency and quality of care than competition between hospitals. Competition is not an end in itself but a mechanism for achieving further improvements in economy, efficiency and effectiveness in the provision of health care. The statutory objectives of the regulator should reflect this, as they do in other industries (such as Ofwat, Ofcom (House of Lords, 2007)).

The White Paper is silent on developing stronger incentives to encourage the emerging coordination across primary and secondary care which can achieve better quality and value in health care. While competition is a feature between such networks in, for example, the United States, the primary drivers of quality and efficiency within the network appear to be more closely related to peer review of performance using better data, coupled with professionalism, and aligned 'intra-network' incentives (Rosen et al., forthcoming; Thorlby et al., 2011; Dixon et al., 2004). Across the NHS there are already many impressive initiatives in this direction, led by clinicians, that need understanding, nurturing and evaluating (Ham and Smith, 2010; Cortese, 2010; Lewis et al. 2010). The government could leave room within its overall national policy for these and similar creative developments drawing both on recent international experience (Casalino, forthcoming) and emerging developments in the NHS (Ham and Smith, 2010; Shaw et al., forthcoming; Ham, 2010; Lewis et al., 2010; Ham, 2009). To help encourage creativity, consideration could be given to removing some national obstacles, by developing the current policy approach to competition and choice, the incentives associated with the prospective payment system for hospitals (Payment by Results), the focus within acute trusts on expanding hospital activity, and barriers to service reconfiguration (Ham and Smith, 2010).

Will the reforms help to increase efficiency to the extent needed to 2014?

The £ 15-20 billion of efficiency savings required to manage within the Spending Review resource allocations equate to productivity growth of between 4 and 5 per cent per annum. This is substantially above the rate of productivity growth in the NHS over the last decade (Phelps et al., 2010). Health Service productivity fell by 0.2 per cent per annum over this decade whilst productivity measured by gross value added (GVA) output per hour worked grew by an average of 2 per cent a year across the economy as a whole.

The reforms, if parliament votes them in, will not take full effect until 2013 – 2014. Until then the Department of Health has estimated that 40 per cent of the efficiency savings needed will come from reducing national tariff prices (which it currently sets, but will not from 2013), 40 per cent through freezing pay rises (the Department of Health sets national pay rates for most staff groups in the NHS) and only 20 per cent through local efforts to for example reconfigure clinical services. Furthermore the recent Spending Review set out national requirements for reductions in management costs across the NHS, the Department of Health and its non-departmental public bodies. Administrative budgets will be cut by 33 per cent in real terms saving £ 1.9 billion.

Locally, managing with lower tariffs and changing clinical services will be a huge challenge. But the challenge will be far greater because of the wide-spread organisational reform, which can mean that services stand still for a period rather than progress (Dickinson et al., 2006). There is clear evidence that organisations distracted by reform can experience some degree of financial and service failure (Audit Commission, 2006). Failure could come in several forms, including a lack of control of expenditure, rushed service changes, or more fundamentally a decline in the quality of care. The latter is the more worrying because quality is less readily measurable than finance, and in the current financial climate there will be much attention to the bottom line. The emphasis in the White Paper on measuring outcomes and developing these indicators is welcome, but these indicators may not signal quickly enough changes in quality.

Even if the broad direction of the reform programme is right – to devolve more autonomy to clinicians – it is not clear that the NHS in England will be able to achieve the efficiencies needed without significant cuts to services, and accompanying public and professional discontent. While public satisfaction levels with NHS care have never been higher, the next few years look among the most challenging ever faced by the NHS.

References

Anderson G and Markovich P (2010) *Multinational Comparisons of Health Systems Data, 2008*. The Commonwealth Fund. www.commonwealthfund.org/Content/Publications/Chartbooks/2010/Apr/Multinational-Comparisonsof-Health-Systems-Data-2008.aspx

Appleby J, Crawford R and Emmerson C (2009) *How Cold Will it Be? Prospects for NHS Funding 2011–2017*. The King's Fund.

Audit Commission (2009) *More For Less: Are Productivity and Efficiency Improving in the NHS?* www.audit-commission.gov.uk/nationalstudies/health/financialmanagement/Pages/20091111moreforless.aspx

Audit Commission (2006) *Learning the Lessons from Financial Failure in the NHS.* www.audit-commission.gov.uk/nationalstudies/health/financialmanagement/Pages/financialfailureinthenhs.aspx

Audit Commission and Healthcare Commission (2008) *Is the treatment working? Progress with the NHS system reform programme.* London: Audit Commission

Baker RG, MacIntosh-Murray A, Porcellato C, Dionne L, Stelmacovich K, Born K (2008) *High-performing health systems. Delivering quality by design.* Longwoods publishing Corporation, Toronto

Bloom N, Propper C, Seiler S and Van Reenan J (2010) *The Impact of Competition on Management Quality: Evidence from Public Hospitals.* The Centre for Market and Public Organisation 10/237, Department of Economics, University of Bristol. www.bristol.ac.uk/cmpo/publications/papers/2010/wp237.pdf

Blunt I, Bardsley M and Dixon J (2010) *Trends in Emergency Admissions in England, 2004–2009. Is greater efficiency breeding inefficiency?* Briefing paper. Nuffield Trust.

Casalino L (forthcoming) *GP Commissioning: Ten suggestions from the US.* Nuffield Trust.

Commission for a High-performance Health System (2006) *Framework for a High-performance Health System in the United States.* Commonwealth Fund. www.commonwealthfund.org/~/media/Files/Publications/Fund%20Report/2006/Aug/Framework%20for%20a%20High%20Performance%20Health%20System%20for%20the%20United%20States/Commission_framework_high_performance_943%20pdf.pdf

Commonwealth Fund (2009) *International Health Policy Survey* http://www.commonwealthfund.org/Content/Surveys/2009/Nov/2009-Commonwealth-Fund-International-Health-Policy-Survey.aspx

Cooper Z, Gibbons S, Jones S and McGuire M (2010) *Does Hospital Competition Save Lives? Evidence from the English NHS patient choice reforms.* LSE Health Working Paper no. 16.

Cortese D (2010) *High Value Delivery Systems: How to achieve them.* www.nuffield-trust.org.uk/events/detail.aspx?id=46&prID=708&year=2010

Department of Health (2010) *Equity and Excellence: Liberating the NHS.* Department of Health.

Department of Health (2005) *Supporting People with Long-term Conditions: An NHS and social care model to support local innovation and integration.* www.dh.gov.uk/prod_consum_dh/groups/dh_digitalassets/@dh/@en/documents/digitalasset/dh_4122574.pdf

Dickinson H, Peck E and Smith JS (2006) *Leadership in Organisational Transition: What can we learn from the evidence?* Health Services Management Centre and NHS Institute for Innovation and Improvement.

Dixon J, Lewis R, Rosen R, Finlayson B and Gray D. (2004) *Can the NHS Learn From US Managed Care Organisations?* BMJ 328: 223–5.

Emmerson C, Crawford R, Brewer M, Brown J and O'Dea C (2010) *Spending Review 2010.* Institute for Fiscal Studies.

Gaynor MS (2006) *What Do We Know About Competition and Quality in Health Care Markets?* Working Paper no. 12301. National Bureau of Economic Research.

Gaynor MS, Moreno-Serra R and Propper C (2010) *Death by Market Power: Reform, competition and patient outcomes in the National Health Service.* Working Paper no. 16164. National Bureau of Economic Research.

Ham C (2010) *Working Together for Health: Achievements and challenges in the Kaiser NHS Beacon programme.* Health Services Management Centre Policy Paper 6. University of Birmingham.

Ham C (2009) *Chronic care in the English National Health Service: progress and challenges,* Health Affairs 28: 190–201.

Ham C and Smith J (2010) *Removing the Policy Barriers to Integrated Care.* Briefing paper. Nuffield Trust.

HM Treasury (2010) *Spending Review 2010.*

House of Commons Health Committee (2010) *Commissioning. Fourth Report of Session 2009–10.* www.publications.parliament.uk/pa/cm200910/cmselect/cmhealth/268/268i.pdf

House of Lords Select Committee on Regulators (2007) UK Economic Regulators Report Volume 1 2006–07. www.publications.parliament.uk/pa/ld200607/ldselect/ldrgltrs/189/189i.pdf

Leatherman S and Sutherland K (2008) *The Quest for Quality in the NHS: Refining the NHS reforms.* Nuffield Trust.

Lewis RQ, Rosen R, Goodwin N, Dixon J (2010) *Where Next for Integrated Care Organisations in the English NHS?* Nuffield Trust.

National Centre for Social Research (NatCen) (2009) *British Social Attitudes 25th Report.* www.natcen.ac.uk/study/british-social-attitudes

Nicholson D (2009) *The Year 2008/09.* Department of Health. www.dh.gov.uk/en/Publicationsandstatistics/Publications/PublicationsPolicyAndGuidance/DH_099689

Organisation for Economic Co-operation and Development (OECD) (2009) *Health Care Quality Indicators Data.* www.oecd.org/document/34/0,3343,en_2649_33929_37088930_1_1_1_37407,00.html

Phelps M, Kamarudeen S, Mills K and Wild R (2010) *UK Centre for the Measurement of Government Activity: Total Public Service Output, Inputs and Productivity.* Office for National Statistics. www.statistics.gov.uk/articles/elmr/elmr-oct10-phelps.pdf

Rosen R, Mountford J, Lewis R, Lewis G, Shaw SN and Shand J (forthcoming) *Integration in Health and Care Services – What are the essential ingredients?* Nuffield Trust.

Royal College of Physicians (2008) *Teams Without Walls. The value of medical innovation and leadership.* Report of a Working Party of the Royal College of Physicians, Royal College of General Practitioners, and the Royal College of Paediatrics and Child Health.

Royal College of Physicians, Royal College of General Practitioners and NHS Alliance (2004) *Clinicians, Services and Commissioning in Chronic Disease Management in the NHS. The need for co-ordinated management programmes.* www.rcgp.org.uk/PDF/Corp_chronic_disease_nhs.pdf

Sassi F and Hurst J (2008) *The Prevention of Lifestyle-related Chronic Diseases: An economic framework.* OECD Health Working Paper, 32. www.oecd.org/dataoecd/57/14/40324263.pdf

Shaw SE, Levenson R, Brandreth M, Connor M and Kissen G (forthcoming) *Old Trafford, New Trafford: Lessons learned from the journey towards an integrated care system*. Nuffield Trust.

Smith J, Curry N, Mays N and Dixon J (2010) *Where Next for Commissioning in the English NHS?* Nuffield Trust and the King's Fund.

Smith JA, Mays N, Dixon J, Goodwin N, Lewis R, McClelland S, McLeod H and Wyke S (2004) *A Review of the Effectiveness of Primary Care-led Commissioning and its Place in the NHS*. Health Foundation.

Smith JA, Wood J and Elias J (2009) *Beyond Practice-based Commissioning: The local clinical partnership. Briefing paper*. Nuffield Trust and NHS Alliance.

Steele G (2010) *Governance and Accountability for Integrated Care: The experience of Geisinger Health System*. www.nuffieldtrust.org.uk/downloads/detail.aspx?id=482

Stremikis K, Davis K and Audet AM (2010) *Health Care Opinion Leaders' Views on Delivery System Innovation and Improvement*. The Commonwealth Fund Data Briefing.

Thorlby R, Rosen R and Smith J (2011) *GP Commissioning: Insights from Medical Groups in the United States*. Nuffield Trust.

Wanless D (2002) *Securing our Future Health. Taking a Long-Term View*. HM Treasury.

Focus On the Patient – The Role of the Patient in Germany's Health Care System

Jens Christian Baas

Abstract

The role of patients in the German health system has changed as they move ever more into the focus. German patients want increasingly to participate in decisions. They want choice and transparency regarding the quality of medical services. The discussion is about partnership rather than paternalism, about evidence in place of eminence.

A demand-driven health care system is based on exactly these informed and confident patients. Therefore, the role of health insurance funds is changing, too. They become important brokers of information and motivators for the promotion of health literacy for mature patients. And they are currently the ones that try to make quality measurable.

In the interest of transparency and the best performance, insurance funds do not need competitive rhetoric but reliable competitive conditions. This is the only way to create a health system in which the individual patient can determine the action and in which quality will become competitive factor no. one.

Zusammenfassung

Der Patient rückt immer stärker in den Fokus des Gesundheitswesens. Zunehmend möchte er in Entscheidungen eingebunden werden, fordert Wahlmöglichkeiten und Transparenz hinsichtlich der Qualität medizinischer Leistungen. Es geht um Partnerschaft statt Paternalismus, um Evidenz anstelle von Eminenz.

Ein durch Nachfrage gesteuertes Gesundheitssystem basiert auf informierten und selbstbewussten Patienten. Deshalb ändert sich auch die Rolle der Krankenversicherungen. Sie werden wichtige Informationsvermittler und Motivatoren zur Förderung der Gesundheitskompetenz des mündigen Bürgers. Und sie sind es, die derzeit versuchen, Qualität messbar zu machen.

Im Interesse von Transparenz und Bestleistung brauchen Krankenkassen keine Wettbewerbsrethorik, sondern verlässliche Wettbewerbsbedingungen. Nur so kann ein Gesundheitssystem entstehen, in dem der individuelle Patient das Handeln bestimmt und Qualität zum Wettbewerbsfaktor Nummer eins wird.

It is not only in legal terms that the insured and patients in Germany bear the bulk of responsibility for their own health. They also shoulder increasingly higher financial burdens in a health care system, whose costs are ever rising due to demographics and the possibilities of medical and technological advancement. Where required, they select for themselves a suitable doctor or clinic, make independent decisions on changing social health insurance funds, and, as patient, *they* decide every day on whether to take necessary medicinal products, whether to attend doctor's appointments, and whether to pursue lifestyle changes.

Based on numerous surveys in 'Trendmonitor Gesundheit' [Monitoring the Trends In Health Care] undertaken by Techniker Krankenkasse, it becomes obvious[1] that a subordinate, passive role in the doctor-patient relationship no longer meets the needs of the insured. Patients wish to play a part in decision-making. They want options, transparency, and information on the quality of health services. It is about partnership rather than paternalism, evidence rather than eminence.

Indeed, the insured and patients are the most important, but frequently forgotten and often underestimated driving force of the medical system. Their need-oriented demand dictates the market. Hence, all players in the health care sector are well-advised to actively and sustainably support the patients' competence. Patients must be in a position to access medically relevant information, to evaluate and implement this, to clearly express their needs and references, and to recognise and critically review quality features to be able to take responsibility for their own health.

In the meantime, social health insurance funds play a decisive role in imparting this health care competence: If necessary, they become the patient's spokesperson, important information intermediaries, and motivators. And it is they who are beginning to make quality in health care both transparent and measurable for the insured.

Partnership Rather Than Paternalism

Even in the 21st century, it cannot be expected from the paternalistically oriented medical sector in Germany to see the patient as a competent partner. The fixed views of people in the specific market of health care, which is still strongly characterised by protective and directive elements rather than by the

---

1   cp. Nebling, T., Fließgarten, A., 2009, p. 86 et seq.

active competence of the citizens, are only slowly changing. Never the less more co-determination of the patients is now possible and they have more means of information at hand. Hence, the Euro Health Consumer Index (an annual measurement standard for Europe's most consumer-friendly health care system ranking more than 30 countries) shows Germany to have a health care system that is not especially patient-oriented. The Germans have excellent access to the benefits of one of the world's most extensive catalogues of services, they rarely encounter waiting lists for medical treatment unlike in Scandinavia and Britain, family members are co-insured under the statutory health insurance, and hardly any German is without health insurance coverage. And yet Germany is annually outperformed by countries like the Netherlands, Austria, and Denmark when it comes to medical outcomes of the system and the use of services: »*Germany – fantastic for access to health, but surprisingly mediocre outcomes. You want healthcare information – ask your doctor!*«[2]

One of the failures of our paternalistic medical system is its absence of transparency when it comes to quality of treatment, particularly in the outpatient sector. As a result, it also lacks reward and incentive systems for good quality. Also symptomatic of Germany is the fact that a patients' rights law has only this year been raised for discussion at federal level.

Other countries have come much further in terms of customer orientation: Denmark is a forerunner in establishing patients' rights and patient information. The Netherlands has more confidence in the consumer sovereignty of its insured in a competition-oriented health care market than has Germany. For many years, America has placed focus on the concept of »Shared Decision Making« and the introduction of »Health Coaches«, the aim of which is to support patients in acquiring health care competence and in making self-determined decisions. At the same time, poor quality standards are also penalised. This means that Medicare, the social insurance programme for elderly and disabled citizens in the US, no longer pays treatment costs that have arisen due to a lack of quality, such as complications after surgery caused by residual foreign bodies left in the patient, air embolisms and blood transfusion errors, or complications like pressure ulcers.[3]

For many years, England's NHS has also carried out long-term monitoring measures with regards to quality, has set quality targets and drawn consequences if standards fail to be adhered to. There was, for example, an impressive reshaping of the NHS with the introduction of so-called »Star Ratings« into the state system: for the first time, organisations providing good quality standards were publicly rewarded, while those failing to meet standards

2   Euro-Canada Health Consumer Index 2009, p. 13
3   Rosenthal, MD, 2007, p. 1573–1575

received sanctions. Only this transparency resulted in managements making greater efforts to look for improved health care solutions and reduce waiting lists.[4]

Patient Focus Is Becoming a Strategy for Company Success

While Germany still lags behind in terms of developments to improve quality transparency, particularly in its outpatient services, the role of citizens in the statutory health insurance market has undergone radical change through the introduction of competition among social health care funds. As consumer, the insured and patient is required to make an independent purchasing decision. In the meantime, changing social health insurance funds is a normal occurrence. Since 1996, one of two people has made use of this right.[5] Apart from the price being a key deciding factor in the appeal of a social health insurance fund (despite the standard contribution, price competition is currently being revitalised through the introduction of unlimited additional contributions), the competing social health insurance funds try to distinguish themselves through high service standards and by responding more effectively to the individual needs of the insured, in so far as permitted under the specified legal framework.

As a customer-oriented company, Techniker Krankenkasse (TK) has at an early stage provided a patient-centred service. And it has done this with great success. Since 1996, the number of its members has doubled. And in 2010, TK was named Germany's best social health insurance fund for the fifth time in a row. The individual customer determines the working practices of all fund employees. This strategic goal lies at the heart of the company's vision. Differentiation is of prime importance. With 300 integrated health care contracts across the whole of Germany for the innovative treatment of heart disease, cancer, psychological disorders, orthopaedic illnesses and many more indications, individually tailored price tariffs are also enjoying growing popularity in the meantime. Through the TK-Meinungspuls [Opinion Pulse], Trendmonitor [Monitoring the Trends In Health Care] (a representative survey among the population to special topics by an independent institute and initiated by TK), and Servicebarometer [Service Barometer] (a representative survey among TK members by the TK department Marketing Planning and Marketing Controlling), the TK regularly carries out surveys among its insured with the aim of identifying their needs and preferences concerning good health care

---

4   Bevan, 2009
5   cp. AOL Bundesverband, Oktober 2006 [Federal Association of Local Health Insurance Funds, October 2006]: Between 1996 and 2006 the changes between social health insurance funds are at 49 per cent.

and service offers. In recent times, a customer advisory board has been set up to support TK through a constructive and critical exchange of ideas on the advancement and new development of products and processes. The Scientific Institute of Techniker Krankenkasse for Benefit and Efficiency in Health Care (WINEG) carries out additional scientific health care research.

In order to further empower the patient's role, TK has developed health care services that enable the insured to obtain and evaluate evidence-based information on health, to practise their own interactive and communicative skills, to recognise and critically review the quality of health services, and to adopt a healthy lifestyle by means of self-management. Health care competence is communicated through the use of both traditional and modern media, such as the Internet, telephone, print media and personal advisors. Participation is voluntary for all the insured. Examples are indicated below:

Innovative information services
- The *TK-Ärztezentrum* [TK-Centre for General Practitioners and Specialists] is an information hotline exclusively intended for TK members. 24 hours a day, 365 days a year, it provides a reliable, supplementary, and always accessible information service, where a total of 100 specially trained medical practitioners are available to offer medical information on almost any field. The service focuses on providing factual information only. No diagnoses or treatment instructions are given. Nevertheless, the provision of evidence-based information allows the insured to prepare for, evaluate, and complement their doctors' visits. The service has been well-received and is met with a high user demand: the TK-Ärztezentrum receives 200,000 calls per year.
- The *TK-Gesundheitscoach* [TK-Health Coach] offers health coaching in both an online and telephone-based context, helping the insured to maintain or improve their health by adopting a healthy lifestyle, or to rebuild their day-to-day independence in spite of serious and chronic illness. Coaching is provided in several areas. For special illnesses such as heart failure or diabetes, telephone health coaching by specially trained nurses is offered. Communication media are also available for smoking cessation, exercising advice, and establishing a useful diet plan. The coach plans an individualised, optimal strategy for the insured, boosts their motivation, and delivers professional feedback on the progress made.
- The web-based, interactive *TK-Patientendialog* [Dialogue with the Patient] is an intelligent expert system that provides the user with individually relevant and evidence-based patient information on illnesses as well as on diagnostic and therapeutic options. In the form of a consultation between the patient and the expert, the system helps to prepare the way for the consultation with the treating doctor and provides support measures

for decision-making on a partnership basis. A total of more than 23,000 people have already used the online TK-Patientendialog, not as a replacement for a doctor's consultation, but as a way of better preparing themselves for such a consultation, or simply as an auxiliary service.

- *Decision support on the early detection of cancer and patient information brochures* are balanced, evidence-based and easily comprehensible patient information services, enabling patients to make informed and self-determined decisions for or against their participation in early cancer detection measures. In addition, the insured have access to around 80 brochures covering a range of medical questions and health care services.

Assessment Tools for Making a Quality Comparison
- The *TK-Klinikführer* [Hospital Guide] is an online hospital search engine, which is intended to help patients in choosing a suitable hospital for themselves. It offers factual information on departments, specialisms, and the specific services of each clinic, as well as information on the quality of treatment. The quality reports of all hospitals have been prepared to be helpful for patients and to aid decision-making. These are supplemented by a traffic light system and information concerning the subjective experiences and impressions of patients, as gleaned from regular satisfaction surveys. 267,000 patients were addressed in 2008. Patient satisfaction values are now available for 624 hospitals and 1,600 departments. New survey findings from by now 350,000 patients and 1,100 hospitals will be made available in 2011. The development of the quality results can be tracked by comparing different survey years. Techniker Krankenkasse has lately also awarded quality seals for clinics that perform above the national average in all five quality fields enquired about in the satisfaction study.
- First study of a *Ärzte-Führer* [Guide on Doctors] in the outpatient sector.
- The *TK-Kursreihe: Kompetent als Patient* [Series Of Courses: 'To Be a Competent Patient'] is a service for all citizens who want to learn how to competently orientate themselves in the health care system. This applies irrespective of the reason for your using the health care system (prevention, check-up & early detection or diagnosis, therapy & rehabilitation), and regardless of whether it concerns your own health or that of someone close to you (e. g. children, spouse our partner, parents or grandparents). As responsible citizens, the insured are encouraged to make informed and self-determined decisions that have a positive impact on their health. They learn how to find, evaluate and use health information, how to have a successful consultation, and how to find and evaluate suitable health care providers.

A demand-driven health care system is based on informed and self-confident patients and insured. This means that in the future, social health insurance funds will not only provide medical measures by means of concluding respective contracts with suitable health care providers. They are already becoming important information intermediaries and motivators for promoting health care competence among responsible patients, thereby unburdening the medical community. And they are also in the process of making quality measurable.

Conclusion

Increasing emphasis is being placed on the patient's role within the health care system.

And this is an encouraging development. Admittedly, the German health care system must further meet the information needs and wishes of the patients in order to better support patients in becoming responsible partners: More transparency on the quality of care, more health care services that reward high medical standards and the participation of the insured, more differentiation and individual options are high on the health agenda of the future. In an effort to achieve this transparency and the best possible service, the German social health insurance funds do not need competitive rhetoric, but reliable competitive conditions: an obligatory political regulation framework that equally applies to all players and replaces short-term reform efforts and interventions in trifles, a uniform supervisory authority, more freedom of contract and financial scope. This is the only way to create a health care system, in which the individual *patient* determines the course of action and where quality becomes the primary competition parameter.

Literature

Bevan, Gwyn (2009), *Ernstgemeinte Leistungsbeurteilungen – Ein Ansatz zur Verbesserung des Gesundheitssystems [Serious Performance Appraisals – An Approach to Improving the Health Care System]*, in: Amelung et al. (ed.), Managed Care in Europe, Berlin
Eriksson, D., Björnberg, A. (2009), *Euro-Canada Health Consumer Index 2009*, FCPP Policy Series No. 61/ May 2009
Nebling, T., Fließgarten, A. (2009), *Wollen Patienten mündig sein? [Do Patients Want to Be Responsible?]*, in: Klusen, N., Fließgarten, A., Nebling, T. (ed.), Informiert und selbstbestimmt, Beiträge zum Gesundheitsmanagment, Band 24 [Informed and Self-Determined, Articles on Health Care Management, volume 24], Baden-Baden

Rosenthal, MD (2007), *Nonpayment for Performance? Medicare's New Reimbursement Rule*, NEJM Volume 357: p. 1573–1575

Chapter 3:
Hospital Sectors in the EU –
Facing Change?

Current and Future Strategic Challenges of German Hospitals

Jörg F. Debatin

Abstract

Hospital-based health care in Germany has evolved from a totally non-transparent and heavily process-regulated system to a competitive market. To survive in such a market, hospitals were forced to consciously define their product portfolios. These should be based on quality, profitability and Unique Selling Proposals. The bases of marketing and sales strategies must lie in providing transparency to the customer, i.e. the patient, regarding outcome quality of health care products.

Zusammenfassung

Das Krankenhaussystem im deutschen Gesundheitswesen hat sich von einem komplett undurchsichtigen und stark prozessbestimmten System zu einem wettbewerbsfähigen Markt entwickelt. Die Krankenhäuser wurden gezwungen, ihre Produktportfolios klar zu definieren, um in einem solchen Markt überleben zu können. Diese Portfolios sollten auf Qualität, Profitabilität und Alleinstellungsmerkmalen basieren. Als Grundlage für Marketing- und Verkaufsstrategien muss die Ergebnisqualität hinsichtlich von Produkten für die Gesundheitsversorgung dem Kunden, d. h. dem Patienten, transparent gemacht werden.

I) Introduction:

Until 2004 health care had remained largely insulated from normal market mechanisms. Rather, health care providers were operating in a jungle of rules and regulations created by bureaucrats and enacted by politicians. Obviously, there are many reasons why health care cannot be considered a »normal market«. First and foremost, health is a very special commodity which should be affordable for all members of a society regardless of their income levels. Acceptance of this paradigm remains the basis for all European health care systems. Unfortunately, the reliance on rules and regulations to assure sufficient quality of health care is not really warranted. In contrast to all other products, regulations governing the health sector only affect the process of

73

administrating health care regardless of outcome. If the same principles were applied to the production of cars, the assembly of brakes in a car would be regulated whereas performance of the same brakes would not be subject to any checks at all. Increasingly patients are becoming aware of this central short-coming of European health care systems.

At the turn of the century it had become clear that insulation from market mechanisms had resulted in rather inefficient health care service structures throughout Europe in general and in Germany in particular. Therefore Germany enacted fundamental health care reform on 1 January 2004 by introducing a DRG system as the basis for hospital service remuneration. Within pre-defined regions the pricing basis was homogenized for all hospital service providers over a period of four years.

This reform changed the business model for all hospitals virtually overnight. The implementation of a DRG-based system introduced market mechanisms based on supply and demand into a very heavily regulated health care market. By basing payment on treating a patient within a defined diagnosis (DRG system) in the setting of a transparent and homogenized pricing system, the element of competition was introduced. Hospitals were forced to consider their cost structures and, more importantly, began to compete for patients. Since prices are regulated within each region, competition was quickly focused on quality. This development has had a markedly positive influence on both the efficiency and the quality of health care delivery in German hospitals.

In the aftermath of this profound health care reform, German hospitals remain challenged by a number of factors. Three crucial elements which must be part of any survival strategy will be briefly highlighted:

II)   *Defining product portfolio:*

In many hospitals most employees are not even aware of their hospital's product portfolio. By in large health care services offered in a specific hospital have developed in a historic sense. While there are variations in the number and type of health care products offered by different hospitals, few providers have consciously decided upon what is offered as part of the existent product portfolio. Rather, portfolios appear to be the results of historic processes based on individual physicians interests and abilities as well as perceived patient needs, expressed by insurance carriers. Frequently, a hospital offers various health care products for no identifiable reason at all.

As a first step in the process of developing any marketing strategy, the currently offered products should be listed. Using portfolio analysis tools each of these products should be analyzed regarding quality, profitability, and future

74

relevance. The assessment of quality and profitability should be based on comparative benchmarking data. Both factors generally relate to volume. Thus, there is ample data illustrating a direct relationship between outcome quality of a particular procedure or operation and the number of times that this procedure is performed within the same hospital in a given time frame. Case volume has also emerged as a direct predictor for cost. Similar to most other products, economy-of-scale effects contribute toward reduced cost also of medical procedures. Put differently: the same procedure becomes less expensive if it is performed more often within the same hospital.

Product portfolios should be consciously defined based on different criteria including quality, cost and 'future relevance'. This is an ongoing challenge which requires hospital administrators to work closely together with leading physicians and lead nurses.

III) *Identifying Unique Selling Proposals (USPs):*

Future relevance of products relates to existent Unique Selling Proposals (USPs) of the hospital offering the product. Each hospital should define these USPs which set it apart from its most direct competitors. USPs can relate directly to the type of patient group served by the hospital (community hospital vs. specialised referral centre), offered medical services (cardiac surgery or organ transplantation), or the quality of care provided. In addition to that, USPs can also relate to aspects of process affecting all products such as a special means of nursing, the implementation of a quality assurance programme or a particularly innovative means of electronically archiving medical patient data.

USPs should be designed to be as defensible as possible. Thus, USPs which can easily be copied by a competitor are of considerably less value than those which will remain truly unique preferably over a very long period of time. However, Unique Selling Proposals should be associated with 'high barriers of entry' for any potential competitor.

For a University Medical Centre the following USPs seem to bear relevance:
1. All products requiring an interdisciplinary approach:
   Since university hospitals will generally be home to more sub-specialists than any other hospital, diseases requiring a multi-disciplinary approach will be treated in a more efficient manner.
2. Complex diseases requiring intensive care:
   Since university hospitals are generally equipped with vast intensive care resources, they should be used for the treatment for the most complex disease entities requiring such services.

3. Ability to adapt to new therapies:
   Since university hospitals encompass research as well as medical care, it should be far easier to implement new medical advances in health care products.

Once defined, the USPs should be checked against those products which have been determined to be both of high quality and high profitability. After all, only those products combining defensible USPs with high medical quality and profitability should be further developed and entered into a future product portfolio.

IV) *Developing a hospital marketing and sales strategy:*

Once a product portfolio has been defined, the hospital infrastructure has to be developed in a manner to strengthen the ability to deliver these products at maximal quality and minimal cost. These efforts should be made transparent to the customer by publishing them on the web. Furthermore, these efforts must provide the basis for any direct sales strategy which, in contrast to most other industries, can only be based on quality and not on pricing. In this regard it is most important to provide transparency regarding the definition of quality. Unfortunately these aspects are not yet regulated in a homogeneous manner. Thus each hospital service provider has to create their own system.

Hence all marketing with advertisement strategies need to focus on information to the patient. Transparency should be provided regarding the quality of the medical products offered. The creation of an attractive and content-rich Internet platform clearly represents a corner-stone in this undertaking. Furthermore, occasional press releases documenting the success of medical treatments should be prepared and distributed into all available channels. Finally, advertisement strategies can also include direct marketing measures such as letters to treated patients outlining progress in diagnosis and therapy regarding their disease. The health care provider should be careful however to respect all laws and regulations governing advertisement in the health care sector in most European countries.

V) *Summary:*

Hospital-based health care in Germany has evolved from a totally non-transparent and heavily process-regulated system to a competitive market. To survive in such a market, hospitals were forced to consciously define their product portfolios. These should be based on quality, profitability and Unique Selling Proposals. The basis of marketing and sales strategies must lie in providing transparency to the customer, i.e. the patient, regarding outcome quality of health care products.

The Impact of Health Care Reform on Quality in the English Hospital Sector

Zack Cooper, Alistair McGuire

Abstract

Theory suggests that under endogenous variable-price regimes, health care reforms which increase competition amongst hospital providers have an ambiguous impact on hospital quality. Hospitals can reduce costs by chiselling on quality. With exogenous fixed-price regimes, on the other hand, health care reforms which increase competition amongst hospital providers can lead to improved outcome quality. There is not a large volume of empirical evidence which can be used to support this theoretical conclusion, but the literature that does exist is indeed supportive. The methods used tend to be similar and reliant on robust estimation procedures and large data sets. To the extent that there are qualifications in this empirical finding it is that the measure of hospital quality tends to be similar and uni-dimensional, e.g. 30-day AMI mortality. Whilst there are justifiable reasons for the choice of this measure, it is associated with emergency admissions and treatment which is difficult to manipulate by the hospital providers. The generalisability of the empirical findings rests upon a belief that there is strong correlation between this dimension and other less verifiable dimensions of hospital quality. If this evidence is accepted, the policy implications appear clear, i.e. that with a fixed-price regime competition can be improved. That this is not found when prices are set endogenously is perhaps an unsurprising lesson.

Zusammenfassung

Grundsätzlich scheinen endogene, auf variabler Preisgestaltung basierende Gesundheitsreformen, die den Wettbewerb unter Krankenhausanbietern steigern, einen strittigen Einfluss auf die Qualität der Krankenhäuser zu haben. Krankenhäuser können die Kosten reduzieren, indem sie bei der Qualität schummeln. Bei exogenen Festpreissystemen können andererseits Gesundheitsreformen, die den Wettbewerb zwischen Krankenhausanbietern steigern, zu einer besseren Ergebnisqualität führen. Es gibt nicht viele empirische Studien, die diese theoretische Schlussfolgerung unterstützen, aber die existierende Literatur bekräftigt diese These. Die angewandten Methoden sind oft ähnlich und basieren auf Schätzverfahren und großen Datensätzen. In dem Maße, in dem es Vorbehalte zu diesen empirischen

Erkenntnissen gibt, neigt die Qualität der Krankenhäuser dazu, gleich und eindimensional zu sein, z.B. Herzstillstand innerhalb von 30 Tagen nach Infarkt. Obwohl es berechtigte Gründe für die Wahl dieser Maßnahme gibt, ist es mit einer Notaufnahme und einer Behandlung verbunden, die von den Krankenhausanbietern nur schwer zu beeinflussen ist. Die Verallgemeinerung von empirischen Studien gründet sich auch in der Überzeugung, dass es eine hohe Korrelation zwischen dieser Dimension und anderen, weniger belegbaren Dimensionen der Krankenhausqualität gibt. Wenn diese Aussage akzeptiert wird, werden die Schlussfolgerungen der Strategierichtlinien klar: Der Wettbewerb kann mit einer Preisfestschreibung verbessert werden. Dass das aber nicht zutrifft, wenn die Preise endogen festgelegt werden, ist vielleicht eine wenig überraschende Lektion.

1. Introduction

Reform of the hospital sector centred around patient choice and hospital competition have been pursued as a means of creating incentives for health care providers to improve their performance and efficiency (Le Grand, 2007). To that end, a range of specific policies designed to increase both patient choice and hospital competition have been introduced in, amongst other countries, England, Denmark, Sweden, Norway and the Netherlands (Bevan et al., 2010, Propper et al., 2006b). A primary concern arising from such reforms is the effectiveness of hospital competition to provide improvements in quality, responsiveness and efficiency. Theory would suggest that if hospital prices are not fixed but endogenously determined and quality is not easily observed or verifiable, then hospitals may react to increased competition for funds by trading off prices for quality, attracting higher volume and funding but producing lower-quality output (Gaynor, 2004). Competition may be introduced but it may not produce the desired effect. Theory also suggests, however, that if prices are set exogenously, increased competition will lead to higher quality, although if provider preferences are sufficiently altruistic, high-quality provision can also occur within a restricted competitive environment (Brekke et al., 2009). Indeed Brekke et al. (2009) show that, theoretically, if altruism is sufficiently high there may be a negative relationship between competition and quality provision. Thus examination of the incentive structures and the environment into which these are introduced is critical.

The British National Health Service (NHS) has always been one of the most centralised health care systems in the world. Funded by general taxation, the UK government has historically had an active role in delivering health care services through centrally run hospitals. However, during the 1980s, the NHS had come under increasing pressure to become more efficient. The response was the creation of a quasi-market in the 1990s that separated purchasers from providers and attempted to create competition on the supply side in England (Enthoven, 1991, Le Grand and Bartlett, 1993). This so-called internal market had at most a limited impact on efficiency, with a major criticism being that, with neither control over the cost nor the quality of provision, hospitals could trade-off cost, quality and outcome to their advantage. The internal market was subsequently abandoned in 1997 with a change in government (Propper et al., 2008, Propper et al., 2004).

The new Blair administration, reacting to concern over access to health care and poor health outcomes in the UK, dramatically increased spending on the health service, and began rolling-out a variety of further reforms, characterised in Figure 1 below, within the English NHS (Klein, 2006). First, the incoming Government set a series of demanding performance targets (primarily involving reductions in waiting times), coupled with so-called performance management programmes (in reality, central direction) to ensure that the targets were met. Then the Government launched a hugely ambitious set of market-based reforms to the English NHS that focused on promoting patient choice and reintroducing hospital competition which were finally implemented in 2005. Unlike previous efforts aimed at establishing an internal market, this initiative relied on patient choice as the mechanism to drive competition coupled with fixed hospital prices for different types of care provision. Every NHS patient in England who needed elective surgery was given a choice of which hospital they attended, with data on different dimensions of hospital quality published to help inform these choices. The core concept was that, given a regime of fixed prices, hospitals would compete for patients and therefore revenue, through improving the quality of care offered. The fixed hospital prices were essentially based on Diagnostic Related Group (DRG) prices for pre-defined case groupings.

Those in favour of hospital competition in the English NHS argued that this would improve efficiency and quality by creating incentives for hospitals to increase their performance or risk losing their market share (Le Grand, 2009). Those against competition argued that the market-based reforms would destabilize hospitals, increase transaction costs and harm patients (Hunter, 2009). A further strand of the competition debate in England were fears that creating a market will harm equity and undermine the traditional 'public service ethos' (Barr et al., 2008). Some critics even argued that the reforms were a threat to the values of the NHS, could lead to inefficiency and would harm equity (Appleby and Dixon, 2004, Barr et al., 2008, Hunter, 2009).

Figure 1. *A characterisation of the English NHS Reforms from 1997 to 2009*

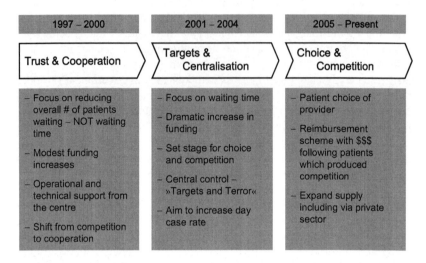

Note: With the recent change in government further reforms, essentially the re-introduction of an internal market centred around individual GP budget holders as funders, and the removal of fixed hospital prices are about to be introduced. It is, at time of writing, too early to evaluate these recent reforms empirically.

This paper assesses whether the introduction of patient choice and hospital competition in the English NHS improved hospital quality, and patient outcomes. It does so in two manners. First we assess the general literature which considers hospital competition and quality, before turning to empirical findings specific to the English NHS. Prior to this examination of the literature however, we consider the conceptual difficulties of measuring competition in this sector.

2. *Issues in measuring competition*

To assess the impact that hospital competition has on clinical quality there has to be an agreed definition of market power. The major challenge being the estimation of the size of the competitive market and the power exercised by individual hospitals (Baker, 2001, Kessler and McClellan, 2000). It is obvious that incorrect definition of the potential market would result in biased assessment of the impact of competition.

In product markets price relationships, in particular own-price and cross-price elasticites, may be examined to aid definition of the relevant market. In the hospital sector this is not relevant as prices, if in fact known, are highly regulated. Typically, investigators calculate hospital market size through concentrating on the definition of geographic area and do so in one of three ways. First, geographic market area may be defined as based on a fixed radius, defined by a largely arbitrary distance that creates a circular market of radius r. Investigators then calculate the degree of competition inside that market. Fixed radius measures have the possibility of both over- and under-estimating the actual size of the market. The shortcoming of such fixed radius measures is that they do not take account of potential demand when they estimate market size. As a result, the fixed radius measures may suffer from urban density bias and overestimate competition in urban areas. However, the advantage of this type of fixed radius market definition is that the market size tends not to be endogenous to any other factors, such as hospital quality.

A second option is to create a variable radius market where the radius r that dictates the size of the market varies according to pre-existing referral patterns, actual patient flows, or hospital catchment areas. For instance, a variable radius r could be set at a length that captures the home addresses of 75 per cent of patie11nts at a particular hospital. Variable radius measures tend not to be as impacted by urban density bias, but some argue that when the radius r that defines the size of the market is based on existing referral patters or hospital catchment areas, the market size they estimate may be biased (Kessler and McClellan, 2000). For example, a high performing hospital may have a larger catchment area than a lower-quality competitor.

A third option is to create a radius that varies according to travel distance. An example of a travel-based radius would be to define radius r as the distance that captures the hospitals within a thirty-minute travel time from a particular patient's home address. Markets definitions based on existing referral patterns may be related to the real or perceived quality of local hospitals, but can suffer from referral patterns reflecting quality. Kessler and McClellan (2000) indeed argue that any estimates of competition that rely on actual patient flows may be biased. Rather than using actual patient flows, they use simulated demand patterns to estimate competition, in essence using actual flows to create an instrumented variable of patient demand. Propper et al. (2004), for example, use travel distance for patients to estimate market size. Propper et al. (2004) argue that their method, based on predicted demand, also mitigates the problems of traditional fixed and variable market measures of competition. However in practice, markets defined using radii derived from travel distances tend to be highly correlated with fixed radius markets. Because the two market definitions produce results which are so closely correlated, they both tend to be affected by similar urban density bias. The key issue with both market definitions is that they require a largely arbitrary definition of the size of the market, such as 30 km for the fixed measure and a thirty-minute travel time for the time variable measure. As such, both market definitions may either over-estimate or under-estimate the true size of the market depending on how the upper boundary of the market is set by researchers.

All three approaches have been applied to the hospital; none are perfect. Each measure has respective strengths and weaknesses and inherent bias. A practical approach in considering which method to employ is to assess the compatibility of the data with the various measures, to trade-off the inherent bias contained in each method by comparing across a number of measures and to explore the use of instrumental variables to overcome any endogeneity.[1]

3. *General evidence on the relationship between hospital competition and clinical quality*

The largest volume of literature assessing the relationship between hospital competition and quality comes from the US (see Gruber, 2006, for an overall review). The bulk of the existing literature has investigated the relationship between competition, prices and capacity and is rather dated and not directly relevant to the English situation (e.g. see Hughes and Luft, 1991, Joskow, 1980, Noether, 1988, Robinson and Luft, 1985a, Robinson et al., 1987, Robinson and Luft, 1985b, Wolley, 1989, Zwanziger and Melnick, 1988). There is a related small, but growing literature in the US that looks directly at the impact of hospital competition on clinical performance. A number of studies consider endogenous price environments and, unsurprisingly, the general finding with respect to the influence of increased competition on outcome quality is ambiguous (e.g. see Gowrisankaran and Town, 2003, Ho and Hamilton, 2000, Sari, 2002).

A smaller number of recent studies on competition and quality tends to the conclusion that, under exogenously determined fixed-priced competition, higher levels of competition generally lead to improvements in clinical performance. Note that the bulk of this US literature on hospital competition and clinical quality examines the outcomes of Medicare beneficiaries and within the timeframe of these studies, Medicare operates an exogenously determined DRG pricing scheme.

Thus Shortell and Hughes (1998) analyse the relationship between in-hospital mortality and hospital concentration and find a small but insignificant correlation. Kessler and McClellan (2000) examine the impact of hospital competi-

---

1 There is a related literature on the specification of patient choice as a determinant of hospital demand which attempts to provide empirical evidence on the reaction of demand to changes in hospital output, including quality characteristics, as a means of quantifying market power. We do not consider this literature here but the reader is directed to Tay (2003) for a useful example.

tion on AMI mortality, the adopted measure of quality, for Medicare beneficiaries from 1985 to 1994. They simulate demand in order to create measures
of competition that are not based on actual patient flows. They find that in the
1980s, the impact of competition was ambiguous but in the 1990s, they find
that higher competition led to lower prices and lower mortality.

Interestingly Gowriskaran and Town (2003) found that competition impacted
Medicare patients and HMO enrollees differently. They found that higher
competition led to a decrease in mortality for HMO enrollees, but that it led to
an increase in mortality for Medicare patients. Others have postulated that this
result stemmed from Medicare rates that were set too low. Shen (2003) also
finds that lower market concentration leads to worsened mortality amongst
Medicare patients. While Kessler and Geppert (2005), using similar method-
ology to Kessler and McClellan (2000), found that competition was not only
associated with improved outcomes in their Medicare population, but it also
led to more intensive treatment for sicker patients, and less intense treatment
for healthier patients who needed less care.

4. Evidence on the impact of hospital competition in the NHS

The vast majority of the English literature on hospital competition is based on
the earlier influence of competition as associated with internal market. Note
that under this set of reforms, hospital prices were not fixed and can be
assumed endogenous. There is wide consensus that the internal market never
created high-powered incentives for hospitals or developed a significant
degree of competition (Le Grand, 1999). Notwithstanding this criticism there
is some evidence that prices fell during the internal market (Propper, 1996,
Propper et al., 1998, Soderlund et al., 1997). Soderlund et al. (1997) also
found that higher competition was not associated with lower quality.

Hamilton and Bramley-Harket (1999) examined the impact of the NHS internal market on patient waiting times and length of stay for hip replacement
from 1991 through 1994/5. Using survival analysis to look at hospital level
data during the internal market reform period, they found that waiting times
for hip replacements fell and so too did patients' average length of stay. They
found that after the internal market was introduced, patients were more likely
to be transferred to another facility, rather than remaining in the hospital
where they had the surgery until they were ready to be discharged home
(Dixon, 2004).

The strongest evidence on the impact of hospital competition on patient quality in the NHS comes from three papers by Propper and colleagues (2004,
2008 and 2010) and one from Cooper et al. (2010). All this work applies dif-
ference-indifference estimation to identify the impact that hospital sector

85

reform has on hospital quality, relying on 30-day AMI mortality as the main quality outcome measure. The estimation procedure defines control and treatment groups and uses common trends affecting both groups over time to identify the impact of the hospital reform on the outcome variable. Thus all these studies consider various aspects of hospital reform, defined as increased competition, on an outcome defined as hospital quality. The dominant quality measure, 30-day AMI mortality, is chosen as, being tied to an emergency treatment and largely associated with in-hospital mortality, it is not easily manipulated by hospital admissions policies. The mechanisms through which AMI mortality may be used as a proxy for general hospital quality are not always made explicit, but hinge around the presumed correlation between the management of AMI treatment and wider hospital practices.

Propper et al. (2004) consider the impact of the internal market, a presumed competitive environment, on hospital quality prior to 1999; that is, they consider a period prior to the fixing of hospital prices. They measure competition using hospital counts within markets defined using a 30-drive times from ward centres. Using hospital level data and controlling for hospital and local area characteristics, they find that the internal market led to a small but statistically significant increase in 30-day AMI mortality, the adopted measure of quality (Propper et al., 2004).

A further 2008 study by Propper et al. (2008) uses hospital panel data and difference-in-difference estimation over a longer time period to see whether more competitive areas had higher or lower AMI mortality over the period 1991–1999. So once again this is a period of endogenously determined prices. Similar to the findings from their previous work, the report that higher competition during periods of competition was associated with higher AMI mortality; i.e. higher competition is associated with lower hospital quality in this dimension. They argue that it is not credible that hospitals deliberately sought to curtail quality in this manner – hospitals did not deliberately worsen 30-day AMI mortality. Rather it is suggested that as the internal market increased competitive pressures, hospital resources were shifted from quality domains that were not fully observable and verifiable such as AMI mortality to those, such as waiting times for elective procedures, that were easily measured and were being targeted.

The introduction of DRG-type prices into the English NHS in 2005/06 fixed hospital tariffs as competition within the NHS was simultaneously strengthened. Two recent studies have used difference-in-difference estimators to examine the impact of this increase in competition on hospital quality using 30-day AMI as the measure of hospital quality. Cooper et al. (2010) find that AMI mortality decreased more quickly for patients living in more competitive areas than that in less competitive areas. Specifically in the three-year period after the reforms were introduced in 2006, one standard deviation more hospital competition was associated with approximately a 1 per cent decrease in AMI mortality. Gaynor et al. (2010) also find a similar impact of the increase in competition on hospital quality, again measured through 30-day AMI death rates, over the period 2003 to 2007. The difference in the data used and precise estimation procedures, Cooper et al. (2010) use individual patient data over a period 2002 to 2008, while the Gaynor et al. (2010) paper considers a shorter period and estimates long-differences contribute as a robustness check, over and above the extensive robustness checks within each individual study, to the finding that increased competition under a fixed-price regime within the English NHS over the period 2002–2008 improved hospital quality.

There is also a small, related empirical literature which considers the impact of increased hospital competition on equity and patient access, the argument being that competition may have a detrimental effect on equality of access for NHS patients. Cooper et al. (2009) consider waiting times for patients having an elective hip replacement, knee replacement and cataract repair over the period 1997 to 2007 in England. They show that waiting times generally decreased as competition increased, and that the variation in waiting times for those procedures across socioeconomic groups was reduced (indeed virtually eliminated). This suggests that equity of access improved over that time period. Cookson et al. (2009) examine the impact of the internal market on equity, measured as the association of between patient deprivation and hospital utilisation. They compare competitive and non-competitive areas, where competition is measured using a Herfindahl-Hirschman (HHI) index in a fixed radius market and also find that there is no evidence that competition had any effect on socio-economic health care inequality (Cookson et al., 2009).

5. *Conclusions*

This short review has confirmed what was to be expected from theory: under exogenous fixed-price regimes, health care reforms which increase competition amongst hospital providers can lead to improved outcome quality. There is not a large volume of empirical evidence which can be used to support this theoretical conclusion but what does exist is rather robust. The methods used tend to be similar and reliant on robust estimation procedures and large data sets. To the extent that there are qualifications in this empirical finding, it is that the measure of hospital quality tends to be similar; 30-day AMI mortality. Whilst there are justifiable reasons for the choice of this measure, it is associated with emergency admissions and treatment which is difficult to manipulate by the hospital providers. It is nonetheless a one-dimensional measure of quality and the generalisability of the empirical findings rests upon a belief that there is a strong correlation between this dimension and other less verifiable dimensions of hospital quality. It is perhaps not too difficult to buy into the belief that if hospitals have good management structures, all dimensions of quality will trend in a similar manner. Other empirical research has indeed found that hospitals with better overall management skills had lower mortality from AMI (Bloom et al., 2010). The policy implications appear clear that with a fixed-price regime, competition can be improved. That this is not found when prices are set endogenously is perhaps an unsurprising lesson. Perhaps unsurprising as at time of writing the English NHS is being subjected to a further round of reform. These reforms aim at pushing competition further by devolving purchasing down to the individual GP level. However this will be supplemented by allowing hospitals to set their own prices. As noted above it is not at all clear, from theory or empirics, that such a move will generate unequivocal benefit.

References

APPLEBY, J. & DIXON, J. (2004) Patient Choice in the NHS – Having Choice May Not Improve Health Outcomes. *British Medical Journal,* 329, 61-62.

BAKER, L. C. (2001) Measuring competition in health care markets. *Health Serv Res,* 36, 223-51.

BARR, D., FENTON, L. & BLANE, D. (2008) The Claim for Patient Choice and Equity. *Journal of Medical Ethics,* 34, 271-274.

BEVAN, G., HELDERMAN, J.-K. & WILSFORD, D. (2010) Changing Choices in Health Care: Implications for Equity, Efficiency and Cost. *Health Economics, Policy and Law,* 5, 251-267.

BLOOM, N., PROPPER, C., SEILER, S. & VAN REENAN, J. (2010) The Impact of Competition on Management Quality: Evidence from Public Hospitals. *CEP Working Paper – 14 February, 2010 Draft.* London, London School of Economics.

BREEKE, K., SICILIANI, L AND STRAUME, O. (2009) Hospital Competition and Quality with Regulated Prices. *CESinfo Working Paper – 2010* CESinfo Group.

COOKSON, R., DUSHEIKO, M., HARDMAN, G. & MARTIN, S. (2010) Competition and Inequality: Evidence from the English National Health Service 1991–2001. *Journal of Public Administration Research and Theory,* 20, 181-205.

COOPER, Z. N., GIBBONS, S., JONES, S. & MCGUIRE, A. (2010b) Does Hospital Competition Save Lives? Evidence From the NHS Patient Choice Reforms. *LSE Health Working Paper – 16.* London, London School of Economics.

COOPER, Z. N., MCGUIRE, A., JONES, S. & LE GRAND, J. (2009) Equity, waiting times, and NHS reforms: retrospective study. *British Medical Journal,* 339, b3264.

DIXON, J. (2004) Payment by results – new financial flows in the NHS. *British Medical Journal,* 328, 969-70.

ENTHOVEN, A. C. (1991) Internal market reform of the British National Health Service. *Health Aff (Millwood),* 10, 60-70.

GAYNOR, M. (2004) Competition and quality in hospital markets. What do we know? What don't we know? *Economie Publique,* 15, 3-40.

GAYNOR, M. (2006) Competition and Quality in Health Care Markets. *Foundations and Trends in Microeconomics*, 2, 441-508.

GAYNOR, M., MORENO-SERRA, R. & PROPPER, C. (2010a) Death by Market Power: Reform, Competition and Patient Outcomes in the National Health Services. *CMPO Working Papers*. Bristol, Bristol University.

GOWRISANKARAN, G. & TOWN, R. J. (2003) Competition, Payers, and Hospital Quality. *Health Services Research*, 38, 1403-1422.

GRUBER, J. (1994) The Effects of Price Shopping in Medical Markets: Hospital Responses to PPOs in California. *Journal of Health Economics*, 38, 183-212.

HAMILTON, B. H. & BRAMLEY-HARKER, R. E. (1999) The Impact of The NHS Reforms on Queues and Surgical Outcomes in England: Evidence From Hip Fracture Patients. *The Economic Journal*, 109, 437-462.

HUGHES, R. G. & LUFT, H. (1991) Service Patterns in Local Hospital Markets: Complementary or Medical Arms Race. *Health Services Management Research*, 4, 131-139.

HUNTER, D. J. (2009) The Case Against Choice and Competition. *Health Economics, Policy and Law*, 4, 489-502.

HO, V. & HAMILTON, B. H. (2000) Hospital Mergers and Acquisitions: Does Market Consolidation Harm Patients? *Journal of Health Economics*, 9, 767-791.

JOSKOW, P. (1980) The Effects of Competition and Regulation on Hospital Bed Supply and the Reservation Quality of the Hospital. *Bell Journal of Economics*, III, 421-447.

KESSLER, D. P. & GEPPERT, J. J. (2005) The Effects of Competition on Variation in the Quality and Cost of Medical Care. *Journal of Economics and Management Strategy*, 14, 575-589.

KESSLER, D. P. & MCCLELLAN, M. B. (2000) Is Hospital Competition Socially Wasteful? *The Quarterly Journal of Economics*, 115, 577-615.

KLEIN, R. (2006) The Troubled Transformation of Britain's National Health Service. *New England Journal of Medicine*, 355, 409-415.

LE GRAND, J. (1999) Competition, Cooperation, Or Control? Tales from the British National Health Service. *Health Affairs*, 18, 27-39.

LE GRAND, J. (2007) *The Other Invisible Hand: Delivering Public Services Through Choice and Competition*, New York, Princeton University Press.

LE GRAND, J. (2009) Choice and Competition In Publicly Funded Health Care. *Health Economics, Policy and Law*, 4, 479-488.

LE GRAND, J. & BARTLETT, W. (1993) *Quasi-markets and Social Policy*, London, Macmillan.

NOETHER, M. (1988) Competition Among Hospitals. *Journal of Health Economics*, 11, 217-234.

PROPPER, C. (1996) Market Structure and Prices: The Responses of Hospitals in the UK National Health Service to Competition. *Journal of Public Economics*, 61, 307-335.

PROPPER, C., BURGESS, S. & GOSSAGE, D. (2008) Competition and Quality: Evidence from the NHS Internal Market 1991–1996. *The Economic Journal*, 118, 138-170.

PROPPER, C., BURGESS, S. & GREEN, K. (2004) Does Competition Between Hospitals Improve the Quality of Care? Hospital Death Rates and the NHS Internal Market. *Journal of Public Economics*, 88, 1247-1272.

PROPPER, C., WILSON, D. & BURGESS, S. (2006b) Extending Choice in English Health Care: The Implications of the Economic Evidence. *Journal of Social Policy,* 35, 537-557.

PROPPER, C., WILSON, D. & SODERLUND, N. (1998) The Effects of Regulation and Competition in the NHS Internal Market: The Case of GP Fundholder Prices. *Journal of Health Economics,* 17, 645-674.

ROBINSON, J. & LUFT, H. (1985a) The impact of Hospital Market Structure on Patient Volume, Average Length of Stay and the Cost of Care. *Journal of Health Economics,* 4, 333-356.

ROBINSON, J. C., GARNICK, D. W. & MCPHEE, S. J. (1987) Market and regulatory influences on the availability of coronary angioplasty and bypass surgery in U.S. hospitals. *N Engl J Med,* 317, 85-90.

ROBINSON, J. C. & LUFT, H. (1985b) Competition and the Cost of Hospital Care, 1972 to 1982. *Journal of the American Medical Associations,* CCLVII, 3241-3245.

SARI, N. (2002) Do competition and managed care improve quality? *Health Econ,* 11, 571-84.

SHEN, Y. C. (2003) The effect of financial pressure on the quality of care in hospitals. *J Health Econ,* 22, 243-69.

SHORTELL, S., AND HUGHES, E, (1988) The effects of regulation, competition and ownership on mortality rates among hospital inpatients, *New England Journal of Medicine,* 318, 1100-1107

SODERLUND, N., CSABA, I., GRAY, A., MILNE, R. & RAFTERY, J. (1997) Impact of the NHS reforms on English hospital productivity: an analysis of the first three years. *British Medical Journal,* 315, 1126-9.

TAY, A. (2003) Assessing Competition in Hospital Care Markets: The Importance of Accounting for Quality Differentiation. *Rand Journal of Economics,* 34, 786-814.

WOLLEY, J. M. (1989) The Competitive Effects of Horizontal Mergers in the Hospital Industry. *Journal of Health Economics,* 8, 271-291.

ZWANZIGER, J. & MELNICK, G. (1988) The Effects of Hospital Competition and the Medicare PPO Program on Hospital Cost Behavior in California. *Journal of Health Economics,* 7, 301-320.

DRG-type hospital payment systems in Europe: the German G-DRG system and English Health Care Resource Groups (HRGs)

David Scheller-Kreinsen, Wilm Quentin, Alexander Geissler, Reinhard Busse

Abstract

The specific design features of DRG-type hospital payment systems remain poorly understood as direct comparisons of payment approaches and incentives of two or more countries are rare. This chapter systematically a) explores the context of DRG-type hospital payment systems, b) outlines underlying rationales, and c) compares the fundamental building blocks German G-DRG system and English Healthcare Resource Groups (HRGs). Our analysis suggests that they are characterised by very distinct design features. Moreover, both systems have developed towards inherently blended provider payment systems, incorporating elements of fee-for-service and global budgets. The incorporation of a quality dimension and a best practice orientation are key future challenges in both DRG-type payment systems.

Zusammenfassung

Die speziellen Gestaltungsmerkmale von DRG-Krankenhausvergütungssystemen bleiben weiterhin schwer verständlich, da direkte Vergleiche von Vergütungsmethoden und Anreizen aus zwei oder mehr Ländern selten sind. Dieses Kapitel
- *untersucht den Zusammenhang zwischen verschiedenen DRG-Krankenhausvergütungssystemen,*
- *zeigt die zugrunde liegenden Erkenntnisse auf,*
- *vergleicht die Module des deutschen G-DRG-Systems mit denen des englischen HRG.*

Unsere Analyse kommt zu dem Schluss, dass sich beide durch sehr spezielle Merkmale auszeichnen. Darüber hinaus haben sich die zwei Systeme zu inhärenten Vergütungssystemen der Leistungserbringer entwickelt, die Elemente der Leistungsvergütung und eines allgemeinen Budgets integrieren. Die Verbindung der Qualitätsdimension und einer Best-Practice-Orientierung ist die Schlüsselherausforderung der Zukunft in beiden DRG-Vergütungssystemen.

1. Introduction

Ever since Medicare adopted the Inpatient Prospective Payment System (IPPS) as the basis for paying hospitals in 1983 in the United States (US), DRG-type hospital payment systems have gradually become the principal means of reimbursing hospitals in most high-income countries (Kimberly et al. 2008). Nevertheless, the motives underlying the introduction as well as the specific design features of DRG-type hospital payment systems vary greatly across countries (Busse et al. 2006, Schreyögg et al. 2006) and remain poorly understood as direct comparisons of payment approaches and incentives of two or more countries are rare (Eggleston 2009).

The introduction of DRG-type hospital payment systems has often been highly controversial, and it is difficult to understand the international success of these systems without being aware of the alternatives. Therefore, this article first provides an overview of traditional hospital payment mechanisms. Subsequently, we introduce the main building blocks of DRG-type hospital payment systems and the objectives and rationales underlying their introduction. Thirdly, the framework of the building blocks is used to guide an analysis of two major European systems: the German G-DRG system and the English Healthcare Resource Groups (HRGs).[1] Finally, we provide an overview of intended and unintended consequences of DRG-type hospital payment systems before concluding with a summary of our findings.

2. Hospital payment

Prior to the introduction of DRG-type hospital payment, countries used three main mechanisms to pay for hospital care: fee-for-service, per diems, and global budgets. Table 1 provides a (simplified) overview of these hospital payment mechanisms, with their underlying incentives concerning four main objectives – even though one may argue about the exact extent of the stated incentives. In addition, the table presents incentives of »pure« DRG-type payment mechanisms. It is clear that each payment mechanism has certain advantages and disadvantages, which are discussed in more detail in the following subsections.

---

1   Analyses covering more countries are conducted in the framework of the EuroDRG project (www.eurodrg.eu), which compares DRG-type hospital payment systems, hospital costs, efficiency and quality of care across European countries and scrutinizes the prospects for a coordinated or even single European DRG system.

Table 1. *Basic payment mechanisms and their supposed incentives in regard to selected objectives*

Payment mechanism	Productivity and number of services	Patient needs (risk acceptance)	Administrative simplicity	Cost containment
Fee-for-service	++	+	-	–
Per diems	+	o	+	-
Global budget	–	–	++	+
»Pure« DRG-type	++ (cases) – (services per case)	- (if insufficient consideration of severity and provided service)	-	o

Notes: ++ / – strong incentive in positive or negative direction; + /- moderate incentive in positive or negative direction, O no incentive in either direction (or dependent on specific details of implementation

2.1 Fee-for-service

Prior to the use of DRGs for hospital payment, fee-for-service (FFS) was the principal means of allocating resources to hospitals in the US. FFS implies that hospitals are paid based on the costs charged per individual patient. This approach was often considered as fair or favourable by providers as long as fees covered their costs. FFS payments provide strong incentives to hospitals to be productive and to do everything they can for their patients. FFS is also good at assuring that those hospitals treating more complex patients are adequately reimbursed. However, FFS may lead to inappropriate or even unnecessary levels of service. FFS payment mechanisms are administratively complex as they require detailed price lists, and registration and billing for all provided services. Furthermore, the only instrument for cost control is the specification of the price list that details the unit payment for each item of service (Street et al. 2007).

2.2 Global budgets

In Europe global budgets were a common approach used to allocate financial resources to hospitals before the introduction of DRG-type hospital payment systems. In the context of global budgets a fixed payment for a certain activity level is agreed at the start of the year. Often global budgets are defined at or adjusted for specialty, though that is not necessarily the case. Global budgets are administratively simple and can effectively contribute to cost containment. However, they run the risk of hospitals not producing sufficient services to meet patient or population needs, hence disregarding patient needs and therefore outcomes. In Europe some countries operate DRG-type hospital payment systems within global budgets in order to control the number of delivered services in a hospital.

2.3 *Per diems*

Under a per-diem regime, applied in some European countries before the introduction of DRG-type payment systems, hospitals were paid a fixed rate for each day a patient stayed in hospitals, often differentiated by specialty. Per-diem payments encourage providers to increase the number of inpatient admissions, to extend the lengths of stay, or both as these strategies result in increased reimbursements irrespective of patient outcomes. Per-diem-based payment systems are administratively simple as they do not require detailed registration of delivered services or coding of diagnoses and procedures. However, they make it difficult for purchasers to control costs as hospitals can try to extend the length of stay of patients beyond necessary levels in order to increase their revenues.

2.4 *»Pure« DRG-type payments*

DRGs often form the basis for case-based payments, i.e. hospitals receive a predetermined payment for a specified diagnosis-related group of patients. »Pure« DRGs refers to the notion that DRGs were originally based mostly on the diagnosis of patients and only to a minor degree on the performed procedures or provided services. Therefore, theoretically, »pure« DRGs provide strong incentives to increase the number of cases treated and to reduce the number of services per case. If they do not sufficiently control differences between patient groups or differences in provided services (within DRGs), payments for highly complex cases are too low whereas payments for less complex cases are too high. Consequently, hospitals could try to select patients that are financially attractive, i.e. those patients whose treatment is less costly than the predetermined payment rate, and avoid the risk of treating more complex patients. Furthermore, DRG-type payment systems are administratively complex as they require detailed and standardised coding of diagnoses and (if used as a source of information) procedures. Concerning costs containment, the effect of DRG-type payments is difficult to predict as it depends on which effect prevails: increasing the number of cases or reducing the number of services per case. In principle, this will also depend on the previous system, i.e. moving from FFS to DRGs can result in cost containment while moving from global budgets to DRGs does not.

In summary, all payment mechanisms provide conflicting incentives for »production of services« and »cost-containment« (Street et al. 2007). Policy makers in Europe have responded to this by combining features of different payment mechanisms: Current DRG-type hospital payment systems do not only consider patient characteristics but also rely on service characteristics to define DRGs. Consequently, hospitals are paid partly on the basis of the services that they provide, which introduces aspects of fee-for-service payments into DRG-type hospital payment. Furthermore, the systems are operated within global budgets, provide fee-for-service add-on payments for specified services or drugs, and per-diem-based reimbursements for patients with exceptionally long length of stay. England and Germany provide a good example for these mixed and highly complex payment mechanisms. Yet, it is essential to understand the main building blocks of DRG-type hospital payment systems before turning to the specificities of the systems.

3. *Main building blocks of DRG-type hospital payment systems*

In general, DRG-type hospital payment systems consist of four fundamental building blocks (Scheller-Kreinsen et al. 2009): (1) a patient classification system (i.e. the DRG system), (2) a data collection system, (3) a price-setting mechanism that defines cost weights or prices per DRG, and (4) the actual hospital payment. Figure 1 illustrates these fundamental building blocks of DRG-type hospital payment systems and the interactions between them. In addition, the figure indicates for each building block a number of methodological specifications and design choices that characterise different DRG-type hospital payment systems.

Figure 1: *Main building blocks of DRG-type hospital payment systems*

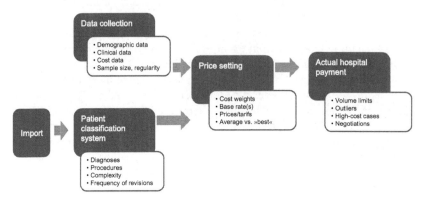

Source: Scheller-Kreinsen et al. 2009 with modifications

The first building block, i.e. the patient classification system, defines »diagno-sis-related« groups of patients, mostly based on diagnoses, procedures, and demographic characteristics, that have (a) similar resource consumption patterns and that are (b) clinically meaningful. By relating patient characteristics to resource consumption, DRGs provide a concise measure of hospital activity or, in other words, they define hospital products. The system has to take into account different levels of complexity of patients. DRG systems can be either imported from abroad (e.g. in Germany) or they are self-developed (e.g. in England).

The second building block, i.e. the data collection system, organises the collection of demographic data, clinical data, and cost data. Clinical data and demographic data are needed in order to group patients into DRGs. Cost data is necessary to ensure costs homogeneity of DRGs. All three, i.e. clinical, demographic and cost data, are used to readjust the patient classification system. Countries differ amongst other things in the size of their hospital samples that they use for data collection, and in the regularity of data collection.

The price-setting mechanism determines resource requirements for treating patients grouped into specific DRGs and sets prices (e.g. cost weights, base rates, tariffs) accordingly. The objective is to give sufficient resources to hospitals enabling them to provide all necessary services. Otherwise, if payment rates are too low, hospitals may cut down necessary services. On the other hand, if payment rates are too high, hospitals are not encouraged to use resources efficiently. Therefore, often information about average costs of treating patients in a sample of hospitals is used to determine relative cost weights or prices for a specific DRG. However, other options exist, e.g. using best-practice tariffs, i.e. costs in those hospitals that achieve higher quality of care or higher efficiency.

The last building block concerns the way in which hospital payment is calculated based on cost weights or tariffs. These mechanisms need to account for the fact that some cases treated in hospitals are significantly more costly than the average case. Therefore, DRG-type hospital payment systems usually require adjustments to the payment rate for these so-called »outlier« cases.

4. *Objectives and rationales underlying the introduction of DRG-type hospital payment systems*

DRGs are often seen primarily as a way to pay hospitals for their services. However, they were developed for a range of different purposes – and they are also used for a much wider range of objectives. These can be grouped into three categories: increasing transparency, inducing efficiency, and supporting the development of management capacity of hospitals.

4.1 *Increasing transparency – performance comparisons*

Central to the original scientific formulation of the DRG concept was the idea common to all classification systems: to condense an extremely large number of items all appearing to be unique (here: hospital patients) to a limited number of groups that have certain characteristics in common (Fetter et al. 1980). The main benefit of such an approach is that it enables certain analyses, which otherwise would not be possible; e.g. the comparison of costs, efficiency and quality. Hence, it is thought to increase transparency about provider performance and resource consumption in an area of policy-making that previously was characterised by extreme agency problems as regulators and payers knew very little about the internal processes of hospitals and had no means to conduct meaningful comparisons. Therefore, conceptually, one of the fundamental advantages is that DRGs offer a framework for an accurate assessment of the costs of treating a given patient, taking account of observable and measurable patient characteristics. Similarly, DRGs can be used to assess other dimensions of performance such quality or efficiency.

4.2   Inducing efficiency – pay and resource allocation

The second motivation behind the introduction of DRGs (used as a payment mechanism) is more ambitious – to allocate financial resources to hospitals. In this role the application and set-up of the DRG system is complex as the aim is not only to reimburse providers fairly for the work they undertake, but also to discourage the provision of unnecessary care and to encourage the efficient delivery of appropriate care. In the context of increasing health care costs, first in the US and later in many European countries as well, DRG-type hospital payment systems fitted well with the paradigm of designing public policy according to general economic principles in order to exert financial pressure and to incentivise efficient resource use, thereby mimicking product markets that produce at marginal costs (Shleifer 1985).

4.3   Supporting the management of hospitals – clinicians accountability

Especially in countries which historically used global budgets or per diems as modes of hospital payment, the management (if it existed) had very little information on what types of services and at what costs clinicians delivered within their wards or departments. Desired or not, DRGs – together with their documentation needs – served to support the development of management capacity within hospitals by enabling them to monitor and assess the work of clinicians systematically.

5.   DRG-type hospital payment systems in England and Germany

The following section first outlines key facts of the hospital markets and the DRG-type hospital payment systems in England and Germany and then continues by scrutinizing design features of the fundamental building blocks outlined above.

5.1   Key Facts of DRG-type payment systems in England and Germany

Key figures of the two hospital markets are presented in Table 2. The main difference between both markets might be the overcapacities on the one hand in Germany versus the waiting lists on the other hand in England. This becomes visible in the number of hospital beds per 100,000 that is twice as high in Germany compared to England. Furthermore, the average length of stay (ALOS) is significantly lower in England, partially due to a higher number of day cases in English hospitals.

Table 2:   *Key figures of the English and German hospital market in 2009*

	England	**Germany**
Expenditures for hospital care/capita (Euros)	1,411	880
Number of hospitals	1,600	2,080
Number of cases	16,806,196	17,519,579
Number of cases per 100,000	32,439	21,334
Average length of stay (ALOS)	5.6*	8.0
Hospital beds	159,386	503,360
Hospital beds per 100,000	308	613
Occupancy rate [%]	85.5	77.5

* percentage of day cases: 32.6 per cent (OHE 2009)
Source: Destatis (2010); Eurostat (2010); Department of Health (2009a)

Table 3 summarises background information on DRG-type hospital payment systems in England and Germany. Overall, DRG-type hospital payment is the single most important payment mechanism in both countries, allocating between 70 per cent and 80 per cent of total acute care hospital expenditures. Health Care Resource Groups (HRGs) and the German (G-DRG) system cover public and private hospitals, inpatients and day cases, and finance recurrent costs of hospital care. In England the system also covers rehabilitation care and includes capital costs. In addition, in the fourth version of English HRGs (HRG4), which came into effect in 2009/10, outpatient care has been included for reporting purposes and for payment of procedures. However, a separate reimbursement system exists for other types of outpatient care. Furthermore, both countries plan to introduce DRG-type payment systems for psychiatric care.

Table 3: *DRG-type hospital payment in England and Germany*

	England	Germany
Patient Classification system	Healthcare Resource Group (HRG)	German DRG (G-DRG)
DRG-type hospital payments as % of total acute care hospital revenues	70%	80%
Applied to	All hospitals treating NHS patients	All hospitals (public and private)
Year of introduction	2003/04	2003
Frequency of revisions	Annual	Annual
Included services		
Inpatient care and day cases	Yes	Yes
Outpatient	Yes (for procedures)	No
Rehabilitation	Yes	No
Psychiatry	No (but planned)	Starting 2013
Included cost categories		
Recurrent costs	Yes	Yes
Capital costs	Yes	No (only some)

Source: Paris et al. (2010) and EuroDRG Consortium (forthcoming).

Both systems have undergone major revisions since they were first introduced for hospital payment in the early 2000s and mechanisms for regular updating of DRG-type hospital payment systems have been developed that ensure the systematic incorporation of changes in service provision (especially the introduction of innovative technologies).

5.2 The patient classification systems: HRG and G-DRG

In England, Health Care Resource Groups (HRGs) were developed by national experts after pilot tests with contemporary US-DRGs had proven incapable of adequately describing English hospital activity. In Germany, the G-DRG system was developed on the basis of an imported version of the Australian Refined (AR-) DRGs. Table 4 summarises the main characteristics of the current versions of DRG systems in England and Germany. The number of DRGs is higher in England (1,400) than in Germany (1,200). In theory, the English system could therefore be able to define more homogenous groups of patients than the German system. Both systems use patient characteristics to classify hospital cases into DRGs, taking into account diagnoses and the age of patients. In addition, the German G-DRG system considers the weight of newborns and mental health legal status as classification variables. Both systems also rely on service characteristics, such as performed procedures or the length of stay of patients in hospitals, and they consider the discharge type (i.e. whether patients were transferred to another hospital) in the classification process. Furthermore, the German system takes into account the duration of mechanical ventilation, whereas only the English system indirectly considers the admission type (i.e. whether patients were admitted as emergencies or electively).

In the English HRG system, base DRGs (called HRG roots) are split into a maximum of three complexity levels if patients within the base DRG are not sufficiently homogenous. In the G-DRG system, the number of severity levels per base DRG is not limited. Thus, base-DRGs are subdivided into as many DRGs as necessary in order to achieve relative homogeneity of resource consumption within each group. In both countries, secondary diagnoses play an important role when determining the complexity level. However, how this information is used differs. In England, a separate list of secondary diagnoses defines complications and comorbidities within a specific chapter. In Germany, secondary diagnoses are aggregated into a cumulative Patient Clinical Complexity Level (PCCL) using a set of exclusion and inclusion rules and considering also demographic characteristics and discharge type.

Table 4: *Classification variables and complexity levels in England and Germany*

	HRG4	G-DRG V.2010
Number of DRGs in 2010 versions	1,400	1,200
Classification variables		
Patient characteristics		
Diagnoses	x	x
Age	x	x
Body weight (newborn)	-	x
Mental health legal status	-	x
Service characteristics		
Procedures	x	x
LOS / same day status	x	x
Mechanical ventilation	-	x
Admission type (i.e. emergency vs. elective)	X*	-
Discharge type (e.g. transfer, regular discharge)	x	x
Complexity levels	3	not limited
Aggregate case complexity measure	-	PCCL**

*   Not explicitly part of the classification algorithm but considered when determining hospital payment
**   PCCL= Patient Clinical Complexity Level

In summary, both DRG systems consider a wide range of variables including patient and service characteristics in the classification process. The English and the German DRG-type hospital payment systems are characterised by a strong procedure orientation. In the G-DRG system procedures have begun to play a more prominent role in the classification algorithm over time (InEK 2009), and in the English HRGs procedures are considered even before diagnoses and in some cases determine payment directly. Consequently, both DRG-type hospital payment systems are inherently blended payment methods as payment depends to an important degree on what hospitals do, thus, introducing aspects of FFS payment into DRG-type hospital payment. In blended payment systems, incentives of one payment mechanism are counterbalanced by incentives related to another payment mechanism. For example, problematic incentives of »pure« DRG systems (exclusively based on information about patient characteristics), such as incentivising reductions in service provision beyond acceptable levels, are offset by considering information about service characteristics, e.g., the type of procedures performed or the duration of mechanical ventilation.

Data collection

Table 5 provides an overview to data collection systems in England and Germany. Both countries collect data about costs of service provision in hospitals: England mandates all NHS hospitals to submit cost-accounting data to a national database, whereas Germany uses data from a sample of hospitals that voluntarily agree to participate in the process of price calculation and follow standardised procedures to do so. Moreover, England and Germany apply different cost-accounting methodologies. In England, hospitals use a top-down costing method, whereas Germany demands hospitals to use a mixture of bottom-up and top-down costing to calculate average costs of treatment of patients (InEK 2007). In Germany, cost data is also used in the process of annual revisions of the DRG system by assessing the homogeneity of costs of hospital cases within DRGs.

In England and Germany, clinical and demographic data are collected from all relevant hospitals. They are used to classify patients into DRGs and to monitor hospital activity.

Furthermore, the English HRG system uses information about length of stay of patients within different HRGs to refine the DRG system. Length of stay data is also considered in the updating process of the G-DRG system, e.g. to calculate length of stay thresholds beyond which cases are to be considered outliers. However, it is not used for the refinement of the DRG system as cost data is more appropriate.

Table 5:   *Data collection systems in England and Germany*

	England	**Germany**
Cost data		
Sample size (% of all hospitals)	All NHS hospitals	250 hospitals (15%)
Cost-accounting methodology	Top down	Mix of top down and bottom up
Data uses	Price setting	Price setting, refinement of DRG system
Clinical and demographic data		
Sample size	All NHS hospitals	All hospitals included in DRG system
Data uses	Classification of patients, refinement of DRG system	Classification of patients, refinement of DRG system

Price-setting mechanism

All DRG-type hospital payment systems aim to set prices at a level that assures adequate payment to hospitals. The objective is to provide enough resources for the provision of all necessary care but to avoid overpayment and related inefficiencies. Table 6 summarises the main characteristics of price-setting mechanisms in England and Germany. In general, the idea of DRG-type hospital payment systems is to use information about average costs of treatment in all or a subsample of hospitals to determine prices. In England, a new development is that the Department of Health has introduced best-practice tariffs for four high-volume HRGs. For these HRGs, prices are no longer set at the level of average costs of treatment but at the level of the most efficient providers (Department of Health 2009).

England and Germany differ in the way they use information about costs to determine prices. In Germany, prices are calculated by using cost weights, which reflect the average costs of patients within each DRG, divided by the average costs of all cases treated in German hospitals. In England, »raw tariffs« are calculated directly based on average costs (or best practice costs) of treatment in all hospitals. Raw tariffs for a given year are usually based on three-year-old cost data but are adjusted in order to account for inflation. In Germany, cost weights are based on two-year-old cost data. In both countries, prices are updated annually.

Table 6:   *DRG price-setting mechanisms in England and Germany*

	England	Germany
Price level	Average costs and (since 2010) best-practice tariffs for four HRGs	Average costs
Payment calculation	Direct (raw tariff)	Indirect (cost-weight)
Applicability	Nationwide (but adjusted for market forces factor)	Cost-weights nationwide (monetary conversion: state-wide)
Time lag to data	3 years	2 years
Regularity of updates	Annual	Annual

Actual hospital payment

Table 7 summarises the main facts about actual DRG-type hospital payment in both countries. As mentioned above, global budgets used to play a prominent role in hospital resource allocation in Europe prior to the introduction of DRG-type hospital payment system, and in many countries they continue to be used to control overall spending. In Germany, for each year the total volume of services that each hospital is allowed to provide (expressed in DRG points) is negotiated. In England, there are plans to introduce a cap on the volume of HRGs to be provided by hospitals.

England and Germany also differ in the way they use prices in actual hospital payment. In England, the actual hospital payment is determined by adjusting the calculated raw tariffs for a market forces factor that accounts for regional variation in wages and other costs of service delivery. These adjustments inflate the raw tariffs by a certain percentage in order to determine hospital specific payment rates. In Germany, calculated cost weights are multiplied with state-wide base rates which are negotiated between the payers and providers.

Furthermore, DRG-type hospital payments are modified by mechanisms similar to per-diem and fee-for-service payments. First, in order to account for cases with extremely long length of stay, both countries provide additional per-diem-based payments for every day of care that patients stay beyond DRG-specific outlier thresholds (Schreyögg et al. 2006). However, only in Germany, if patients are discharged much earlier than the average for a specific DRG, payment is reduced by DRG-specific deductions. Second, both countries have introduced mechanisms that ensure hospitals are rewarded for additional efforts related to the provision of certain high-cost services. In England, chemotherapy, radiotherapy, renal dialysis, high-cost drugs, devices, etc. are reimbursed separately as patients can be assigned to additional »unbundled« HRGs for these services. For each unbundled HRG, hospitals receive additional payments, much like in a fee-for-service system. In Germany, similar mechanisms, i.e. supplementary payments, exist for a similar range of activities. Third, both systems have developed mechanisms to provide additional payments for certain innovative technologies (including drugs) when they are not yet adequately reimbursed through the general DRG-type hospital payment system.

Table 7: *DRG-type hospital payment in England and Germany*

	England	**Germany**
Macro-level price/ volume control	No (plans exist for volume cap)	Yes
Adjustments to price	Raw tariffs adjusted for market forces factor	Monetary conversion of cost weights using state-wide base rates
Per-diem-based outlier adjustments	Long stay: Yes Short stay: No	Long Stay: Yes Short Stay: Yes
Payments for specific high-cost services	Unbundled HRGs for e.g.: Chemotherapy Radiotherapy Renal dialysis Diagnostic imaging High-cost drugs	Supplementary payments for e.g.: Chemotherapy Radiotherapy Renal dialysis Diagnostic imaging High-cost drugs
Innovation-related additional payments	Yes	Yes

6. Effects of DRG-type hospital payment systems

Table 8 summarises intended and unintended theoretical effects of DRG-type hospital payment systems on quality and efficiency.

Table 8: *Intended and unintended effects of DRG-type hospital payment*

Incentives of DRG-type hospital payment	Intended (+) and unintended (–) effects
1. Reduce costs per patient	**Reduce length of stay** + optimize internal care pathways + transfer to other providers: improve coordination/integration with other providers – transfer of unprofitable cases (»dumping«) – inappropriate early discharge (»bloody discharge«)
	Reduce or replace services provided + avoid unnecessary services – withhold necessary services (»skimping«) –/+ replace high-cost services by alternatives (labour/capital)
	Select patients + specialise on patients for which the hospital has a competitive advantage – select low-cost patients within DRGs (»cream-skimming«)
2. Increase number of patients	**Improve reputation of hospital** + improve quality of services – focus efforts exclusively on measurable areas
	Change admission rules – split care episodes into multiple admissions – admit patients for unnecessary services
3. Increase revenue per patient	**Change coding practice** + improve coding of diagnoses and procedures – attempt to classify patients into higher paying DRGs (»up-coding«)
	Change practice patterns – provide services that lead to reclassification of patients into higher-paying DRGs (»gaming«)

On the one hand, DRG-type hospital payment incentivises hospitals to reduce the number of unnecessary services and to optimize the processes of care, which could improve quality and efficiency. On the other hand, hospitals may be tempted to reduce costs by reducing quality.

The effects of DRG-type hospital payment systems on quality, costs, and efficiency were also assessed empirically in England (Farrar et al. 2007, Audit Commission 2008, Farrar et al. 2009) and Germany (Böcking et al. 2005, Hensen et al. 2008, Sens et al. 2009, Fürstenberg et al. 2010), but the results remain inconclusive. In the European context, where, in contrast to the US, DRGs did not replace FFS but global budgets, the effects on hospital costs, average length of stay (LOS) and quality seem to be hard to track empirically.

Nevertheless, most countries are aware of the potentially negative consequences of DRG-type hospital payment systems on quality. Nevertheless, they rarely explicitly adjust payments for quality. Unlike in the US (McNair et al. 2009), where hospitals are no longer paid for certain hospital-acquired conditions, European diagnosis coding systems do not differentiate between diagnoses that were present on admission and those acquired during the hospital stay. This limits their capacity to use diagnosis documentation to define quality indicators and to link payment accordingly.

Nevertheless, England and Germany have introduced measures to deal with potential adverse quality effects. Both systems financially penalise hospitals if patients are readmitted for the same problem within 30 days after discharge. For these patients, hospitals do not receive a second DRG-type payment but are reimbursed through the original DRG. In addition, the introduction of the G-DRG system in Germany was accompanied by regulatory measures such as mandatory quality reports for hospitals, external quality assurance programmes, and minimum volume thresholds (Busse et al. 2009).

In England, the Commissioning for Quality and Innovation (CQUIN) payment framework allows primary care trusts to link a specific modest proportion of providers' income (agreed nationally) to the achievement of realistic locally agreed goals. In 2010–2011, primary care trusts can withhold up to 1.5 per cent of the value of provider contracts if they fail to meet the agreed quality standards (e.g., process indicators or patient satisfaction).

7. *Conclusion: challenges and constraints*

Conceptually, DRGs are clearly attractive for policy makers as they introduce the means to compare hospital performance and resource use. Additionally, in their more ambitious role as resource-allocation instruments, they can induce market-like financial pressure in a sector of health care that was previously sheltered from competitive pressure. As outlined, great care needs to be paid to technical details and operationalisation to a) allow for meaningful performance comparisons and b) incentivise hospitals in line with societal objectives. Our analysis suggests that policy makers in England and Germany attempt to do so by developing inherently blended approaches towards hospital payment, adopting elements of FFS, global budgets, and DRG-type hospital payment systems. Moreover, our analysis shows that the incorporation of quality adjustments and best-practice orientation, rather than comparisons against the average, are key future challenges in both DRG-type payment systems.

Acknowledgements

The findings presented in this paper were generated in the context of the project 'EuroDRG – Diagnosis-related groups in Europe: towards efficiency and quality' (www.eurodrg.eu), which is funded by the European Commission under the Seventh Framework Programme.

References

Audit Commission (2008) The Right Result? Payment by Results 2003–07, Audit Commission for local authorities and the National Health Service in England: London.
Böcking W, Ahrens U, Kirch W, Milakovic M (2005) First results of the introduction of DRGs in Germany and overview of experience from other DRG countries. Journal of Public Health, 13: 128-137.
Busse R, Schreyögg J, Smith PC (2006) Hospital case payment systems in Europe. Health Care Management Science, 9, 3: 211-13.
Busse R, Nimptsch U, Mansky, T (2009) Measuring, Monitoring, And Managing Quality in Germany's Hospitals. Health Affairs, 28, 2: 294-304.
Department of Health (DoH) (2009a) Departmental Report 2009. Department of Health: London.
Department of Health (DoH) (2009b) Payment by Results in 2010–11: letter from David Flory, Director General. NHS Finance, Performance and Operations, Department of Health: London.
DESTATIS (2010) Krankenhausstatistik 2009 (vorläufige Ergebnisse). Statistisches Bundesamt Deutschland: Wiesbaden
Eggleston K (2009) Provider payment incentives: international comparisons. International Journal of Health Care Finance and Economics, 9: 113-115.
EuroDRG Consortium (forthcoming) EuroDRG Country reports – Germany, England. to be published in 2011.

Eurostat (2009) Eurostat statistical database: collection public health – health care expenditures 2008. Statistical Office of the European Communities (Eurostat): Luxembourg.

Farrar S, Sussex J, Yi D, Sutton M, Chalkley M, Scott T, Ma A (2007) National Evaluation of Payment by Results, University of Aberdeen: Aberdeen.

Farrar S, Sussex J, Yi D, Sutton M, Chalkley M, Scott T (2009) Has payment by results affected the way that English hospitals provide care? Difference-in-differences analysis. BMJ, 339: b3047.

Fetter J, Shin Y, Freeman JL, Averill RF, Thompson JD (1980) Case Mix Definition by Diagnosis-Related Groups. Medical Care, 18, (2 Suppl.): 1-53.

Fürstenberg T, Zich K, Nolting H, Laschat M, Klein S, Häussler B. (2010) G-DRG impact evaluation, Final report of the first research cycle (2004–2006). IGES Institut & Institut für das Entgeldsystem in Krankenhaus (InEK).

Hensen P, Beissert S, Bruckner-Tuderman L, Luger TA, Roeder N, Müller ML (2008) Introduction of diagnosis-related groups in Germany: evaluation of impact on inpatient care in a dermatological setting. European Journal of Public Health, 18, 85-91.

Institut für das Entgeltsystem im Krankenhaus gGmbH (InEK) (2007) Kalkulation von Fallkosten, Handbuch zur Anwendung in Krankenhäusern. Dt. Krankenhaus-Verl.-Ges: Düsseldorf.

Institut für das Entgeltsystem im Krankenhaus gGmbH (InEK) (2009) German Diagnosis Related Groups Version 2010. Definitionshandbuch Kompaktversion Band 1. InEK: Siegburg.

Kimberly JR, Pouvourville G de, D'Aunno TA (2008) The globalization of managerial innovation in health care. Cambridge University Press: Cambridge.

McNair PD, Luft HS, Bindman AB (2009) Medicare's policy not to pay for treating hospital-acquired conditions: the impact. Health Affairs, 28, 5: 1485-93.

Office of Health Economics (OHE) (2009) Compendium of Health Statistics. Office of Health Economics: London.

Paris V, Devaux M, Wei L (2010) Health Systems Institutional Characteristics: A Survey of 29 OECD Countries. OECD Health Working Papers No. 50, OECD Publishing: Paris.

Scheller-Kreinsen D, Geissler A, Busse R. (2009) The ABC of DRGs. Euro Observer 2009, 11: 1-5.

Schreyögg J, Stargardt T, Tiemann O, Busse R (2006) Methods to determine reimbursement rates for diagnosis related groups (DRG): a comparison of nine European countries. Health Care Management Science, 9, 3: 215-23.

Sens B, Wenzlaff P, Pommer G, von der Hardt H (2009) DRG-induzierte Veränderungen und ihre Auswirkungen auf die Organisationen, Professionals, Patienten und Qualität. Zentrum für Qualität und Management im Gesundheitswesen, Einrichtung der Ärztekammer Niedersachsen: Hannover.

Shleifer A (1985) A Theory of Yardstick Competition. RAND Journal of Economics, 16, 3: 319-27.

Street A, Vitikainen K, Bjorvatn A, Hvenegaard A (2007) Introducing activity-based financing: a review of experience in Australia, Denmark, Norway and Sweden. CHE Research Paper 30, Centre for Health Economics: York.

Chapter 4:
Providing Health Care to Patients in Europe –
Threat or Opportunity for Domestic Health
Care?

EU Cross-Border Survey 2010 – Quality, Service and Satisfaction

Caroline Wagner, Anne-Katrin Meckel, Frank Verheyen

Abstract

In 2008 TK realised that it would be necessary to learn more about the extent and nature of usage of EU cross-border care among the insurants. In this paper we describe the development of the three EU cross-border surveys 2008, 2009 and 2010 and their different objectives as well as findings. The insurants were asked about their experiences and needs in the context of receiving planned or unplanned medical care in other EU member states. In the current two surveys of 2010 carried out by WINEG we have also asked insurants without experience in order to evaluate their attitudes and the future potential concerning EU cross-border care. The aim has been to generate results to further improve the benefit and service provision of TK in this area. There has been a lot of policy debate concerning this topic, but empirical data are rare. Therefore the gained published data have also been used by health policy and health academics to add facts to the further discussion.

Zusammenfassung

Die TK erkannte 2008, dass es notwendig ist, mehr über das Ausmaß und die Besonderheiten der Inanspruchnahme von EU-Auslandsleistungen durch ihre Versicherten zu erfahren. In diesem Beitrag beschreiben wir die Entwicklung der drei Europabefragungen von 2008, 2009 und 2010 mit ihren unterschiedlichen Fragestellungen und Ergebnissen. Die Versicherten wurden zu ihren Erfahrungen und Bedürfnissen bezüglich geplanter und ungeplanter Behandlungen im EU-Ausland befragt. In den zwei aktuellen Befragungen von 2010, die das WINEG derzeit auswertet, haben wir auch Versicherte ohne diese Erfahrungen kontaktiert. Auf diese Weise soll ihre Einstellung zu EU-Auslandsleistungen und damit das zukünftige Nachfragepotential analysiert werden. Das Ziel aller Befragungen war es, Ergebnisse zu generieren, die zur Weiterentwicklung des Versorgungs- und Serviceangebotes der TK in der grenzüberschreitenden Versorgung relevant sind. Über das Thema wird politisch viel diskutiert, empirische Daten sind jedoch eher selten. Aus diesem Grund sind die publizierten gewonnenen Daten auch von Gesundheitspolitikern und Wissenschaftlern bereits genutzt worden, um der weiteren Diskussion Fakten hinzuzufügen.

In 1998, the European Court of Justice ruled in its Kohll and Decker decisions that health services provided in other EU member states on a remunerated basis constitute services as defined in the EU Treaty. These and later decisions[1] were new and unique. They set the first milestones in EU cross-border care.

Germany was the first EU member state to implement the decisions of the European Court of Justice on patient mobility in national law by passing the Health Modernisation Act of 1 January 2004. Under this act, members of the statutory health insurance system with residence in Germany may claim inpatient and outpatient treatment in other EU member states. From 1 January 2007 this regulation was extended to all states to which the enactment European Economic Community (EEC) 1408/71[2] applies. This covers all member states of the EU, the European Economic Area (EEA) and Switzerland. Iceland, Liechtenstein and Norway are also included as a result of the EEA's agreement with the member states of the European Free Trade Association (EFTA). In these states German patients can claim outpatient and inpatient treatment to which they would be entitled in their own country in any other EU member state without prior permission. Inpatient treatments, though, are subject to prior permission. In both cases, the costs must generally be reimbursed up to the amount which would be reimbursed in the patient's home state if the domestic preconditions are fulfilled.

Since 2004 the legislation allows the statutory health insurance funds to directly enter into contracts with care providers in other EU member states. Techniker Krankenkasse (TK) has at an early stage started to observe the trend of EU cross-border care and consequently provided its insurants with planned EU cross-border health care within an ordinance settlement before the rule was implemented into German law. Moreover, TK has early started concluding direct selective contracts with health service providers in other EU member states for its insurants. The main motives for doing this are to spare insurants the need to pay the services up-front, to relieve the insurants of bureaucratic burden of a protracted reimbursement procedure and to offer the insurants high-quality treatment with German-speaking personnel round the clock. Today, this TK Europe Service encompasses 88 contracted clinics: nine in the Netherlands, four in Belgium, eight in Austria and 67 in Italy. In addi-

---

1   See particularly European Court of Justice (28 April 1998); European Court of Justice (12 July 2001); European Court of Justice (13 May 2003); European Court of Justice (16 May and 15 June 2006).
2   Council Regulation (EEC) No. 1408/71 on the application of social security schemes to employed persons, to self-employed persons and to members of their families moving within the Community.

tion, there are 28 contracts with health and spa institutions: five in Austria, eight in Italy, five in the Czech Republic, six in Hungary, two in Poland and two in Slovakia.

Development of the TK EU Cross-Border Care Studies 2008, 2009 and 2010

In 2000 and 2003, TK has carried out smaller surveys about patient mobility in Europe. The focus of those surveys was the expectations of the members, regardless of actual experiences with EU cross-border health care. Increasing patient mobility and the emergence of the European health care market have been leading to rising use of EU cross-border treatments.[3] Although there is much political discussion on the cross-border utilisation of the European health care market, there have been virtually no empirical investigations to date to determine the extent of actual demand. Therefore in 2008 TK decided to investigate how large the demand for EU cross-border care was amongst the members and what its characteristics are.

The crucial finding was the surprisingly strong increase of TK members receiving planned treatment in other EU member states in the total number of TK members with EU cross-border treatments. In addition to acute and emergency cases, which occur on holiday or during business trips, there is a growing group of patients who increasingly undertake research into their options of being treated in other EU member states in a targeted manner and make use of this option. In 2003, for example, planned treatment and health tourism had not yet begun to play a role: in a TK survey of a sample of 2,100 members, fewer than 7 per cent indicated that they had received planned treatment in another EU member state. In contrast, in the first EU cross-border care study 2008 the proportion of TK members with planned treatments amounted already 40 per cent.[4]

Consequently, the TK Survey on EU Cross-Border Care 2009 focused on the characterisation of the demand for planned treatments as opposed to the demand for unplanned treatments, i.e. acute and emergency cases. This was done in order to identify the different experiences and needs of the TK members according to the respective treatment type.

TK members who are treated on an unplanned basis are a relatively heterogeneous group of patients. In contrast to this, TK members receiving planned treatment in other EU member states can be identified by specific socio-demographic characteristics, diseases, types of treatment and motives. They require different advice and timescales. Because of the element of chance

---

3   See Techniker Krankenkasse (ed.) (2008); Techniker Krankenkasse (ed.) (2009)
4   See Techniker Krankenkasse (ed.) (2003)

involved in acute or emergency treatment, a vast range of TK members are affected here, whose need for advice occurs very rapidly and is very short-term.

TK members receiving planned treatment require more detailed advice over a longer period before availing themselves of the EU cross-border care option. Despite this, the majority still choose their service providers on the basis of recommendations from friends with experience of these services, from their tour guide or from the hotel as well as from their own Internet research. In this regard, there is a demand for TK to provide its members with more support. Furthermore the TK survey on EU cross-border care 2009 has shown that the two key reasons for opting specifically for cross-border treatment in another EU member state are to save money and to combine treatment with a holiday. The latter reflects the trend towards health care tourism even among TK members. The vast majority of the members involved are senior members over the age of 60. TK would like to provide this group of members with an even greater level of professional advice on their way to the European health care market to avoid quality risks and ensure a high level of service concerning the EU cross-border treatment. Therefore the new TK EU cross-border survey 2010 was carried out which concentrated on analysing the experiences of TK members in health care systems of other EU member states concerning quality, service and satisfaction with the cross-border treatment.

TK Survey on EU Cross-Border Care 2008[5]

A study of the EU commission showed that a total of 5 per cent of the German population (four million people) underwent medical treatment in other EU member states.[6] With hardly any other empirical investigations concerning this subject, TK saw the need and implemented the first EU cross-border survey to get specific information on the actual utilisation of medical services at the level of TK, the statutory health insurance system and Germany as a whole.[7]

34,000 TK members were contacted for this survey. The unusually high response rate of 35 per cent demonstrated once again the importance of a European health market and the people´s interest in medical treatment in other EU member states. For the first time, TK had the possibility to specifically survey members who had previously received cross-border medical treatment and applied for cost reimbursement.

5　Unless indicated otherwise, all numbers in this paragraph taken from Techniker Krankenkasse (ed.) (2008).
6　See European Commission / The Gallup Organization (2007), page 7.
7　See Klusen, N. (2008), page 4-5.

Being aware that the TK members who were taking part in the survey are not representative for the respective populations, the results were extrapolated to the level of TK, the statutory health insurance system and Germany as a whole. Despite this deficit this was done to get at least a rough idea how large the demand on these levels is. 34,000 members constitute more than one per cent of all TK members. Extrapolated to the statutory health system, at least 420,000 members, and extrapolated to Germany as a whole, at least 680,000 people received medical treatment in other EU member states. 96 per cent of those questioned TK members did not consider the quality of the treatment to be worse than received treatment in the German health care system. 33 per cent said they were highly satisfied and 37 per cent were satisfied with the quality of the cross-border treatment.

Naturally enough, countries in which medical treatment (planned and unplanned in total) was sought most frequently were the popular holiday destinations Spain, Austria and Italy. They were followed by the Czech Republic, Poland, France, Switzerland and Hungary. Thus including those Eastern European countries in which a conspicuously large volume of health services are utilised for economic reasons.

Table 1: *EU Cross-Border Treatments by Countries*

Country	TK	Statutory health insurance	German Population
Spain	6,595	81,347	131,872
Austria	5,258	64,852	105,132
Italy	4,284	52,833	85,648
Czech Republic	3,312	40,849	66,222
Poland	3,126	38,559	62,508
France	2,077	25,623	41,538
Switzerland	1,923	23,720	38,453
Hungary	1,900	23,438	37,996
Other countries	5,525	68,129	110,445

Source: See Techniker Krankenkasse (ed.) (2008)

According to the information provided by the TK members being questioned in the survey, around 40 per cent of the EU cross-border treatments were planned. The remaining 60 per cent were necessitated by acute or emergency cases. This is a total of 13,564 members of TK who received planned medical treatments in another EU member state. Being aware of the deficits in extrapolating mentioned earlier, this would amount to a figure of at least 167,000 members for the statutory health insurance system and at least 271,000 people (European Commission estimation: a maximum of one million people)[8] in the German population at large. These numbers show that insured people who specifically sought cross-border medical care in another EU member state, but who do not live or work there, constitute an extremely important group in the European market for health services. To be able to adapt to the special needs of those TK members, it is necessary for TK to know the reasons and motives for a planned treatment.

The most important motives for planned treatments in other EU member states in 2007 were with 14 per cent the greater comfort compared with Germany and with 13 per cent the savings on treatments for which a co-payment is required in Germany, e.g. dental work. They were followed by the utilisation of new treatment methods, the specific selection of treatments not acknowledged by orthodox medicine in Germany and the utilisation of certain health care facilities with which TK has special contractual relations. Planned visits to European specialists, medical practitioners of TK members' trust who are based in other EU member states and special clinics in border regions were further reasons for a planned treatment.

Figure 1: *Reasons for Planned EU Cross-Border Treatments*

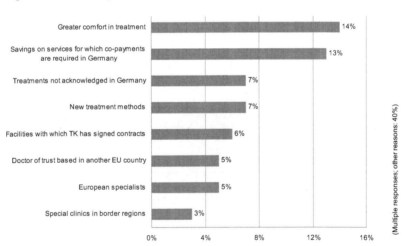

Source: See Techniker Krankenkasse (ed.) (2008), n = 4,777

---

8   See European Commission / The Gallup Organization (2007), page 7.

118

A growing trend in favour of planned treatments was indicated by the break-down of illnesses. 30 per cent of all illnesses comprised (chronic) conditions of the joints and back. This contrasts with the results of the former survey in 2003, in which accident-induced injuries accounted for 25 per cent. Thus, at 14 per cent, acute and emergency situations caused by accidents (open wounds, fractures, burns, poisoning) had declined significantly in importance. This also applied to acute illnesses of the respiratory organs (colds, flu, pneumonia), whose share also contracted from 23 per cent in 2003 to 11 per cent in 2007. One tenth of those asked suffered from dental problems (11 per cent), although not every treatment is likely to have been planned. Cardiovascular problems accounted for 10 per cent.

Figure 2:   *Satisfaction with the TK European Service*

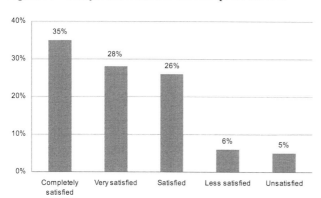

Source: See Techniker Krankenkasse (ed.) (2008), n = 247

To ensure high-quality and unbureaucratic health care in border regions in other EU member states, during vacations and for planned medical treatment, TK has had contracts with clinics for its members since 2004. This service is provided in cooperation with AOK – die Gesundheitskasse and covers the Netherlands, Belgium, Austria and Italy. Until today, contracts were also signed with clinics in the Czech Republic and Poland. Already 20 per cent of the TK members taking part in the survey were aware of TK European Service, even though it was still in the process of being set up. The approval rates were considerable: 35 per cent were highly satisfied and 28 per cent were very satisfied with the quality of the treatment received at the clinics with which contracts have been signed.

EU cross-border treatment poses all different kinds of challenges to health policy. In 2008, the lack of information, financial risks, high dissatisfaction with the cost-reimbursement principle, doubts concerning the quality of the provided medical care, doubts concerning the liability and communication difficulties were the main barriers for the utilisation of cross-border EU medical services. For greater patient safety in the utilisation of cross-border EU medical services, a more active national shaping of EU health policy was needed.

TK Survey on EU Cross-Border Care 2009[9]

The TK survey on EU cross-border care 2009 showed that a constantly growing number of people received planned medical treatment in another EU member state. Reasons for this trend are the emergence of a European health care market and an increasing patient mobility. To enhance the range of services, advice and care options for this specific group of members, TK set the focus of this survey on gaining specific knowledge about the socio-demographic characteristics, the types of illnesses and treatment, motives and needs of those persons, who sought for EU cross-border treatment.[10]

A total of 47,037 questionnaires with 42 questions were sent out in May 2009. All TK members (not TK insurants, i.e. excluding dependent family insurants), 18 years and older, who had at least one medical treatment in another EU member state in 2008 were surveyed. Every treatment, whether it was planned or unplanned, outpatient or inpatient, in all countries where the social security agreement as a result of EEC Regulation 1408/71[11] applies, was considered in the survey. A response rate of 35 per cent, just as high as the response rate in the survey 2008, showed once again the high interest of TK members in medical treatments in other EU member states. After having taken quality control measures, a data set of 15,540 questionnaires, i.e. 29,884 treatments, remained and were verified to be representative for TK insurants. The impact of the results were then discussed with an expert panel, comprised of Prof. Dr med. Reinhard Busse, MPH FFPH, Health Care Management, Technische Universität Berlin; Jeni Bremner, Director of the European Health Management Association (EHMA), Brussels.

The aim of this survey was to answer the three following main questions:

• What influences German patients to cross borders in order to receive planned medical treatment in other EU health care systems?

9   Unless indicated otherwise, all numbers in this paragraph taken from Techniker Krankenkasse (ed.) (2009).
10   Wagner C., Linder R. The Demand for EU Cross-Border Care: An Empirical Analysis. Journal of Management in Health Care 2010; 2(3).
11   Council Regulation (EEC) No. 1408/71 on the application of social security schemes to employed persons, to self-employed persons and to members of their families moving within the Community.

- What distinguishes this group of patients?
- And how many people actually opt to do this?

Of the total number of TK members surveyed, more than two-thirds had to receive treatment in other EU member states due to acute and emergency cases; 40 per cent opted quite consciously to receive EU cross-border treatment, enquired about these options and planned treatment in advance. An analysis of the number of cases instead of the number of TK members results in a much larger basic population, since there are members who have caused several cases of treatments. Of these 29,884 cases of treatments more than half (16,476) were planned and only 45 per cent were unplanned. These results shows that in EU cross-border care, selective treatments now play a more important role than acute and emergency treatments.

Figure 3:   *TK Members with EU Cross-Border Treatments by Age*

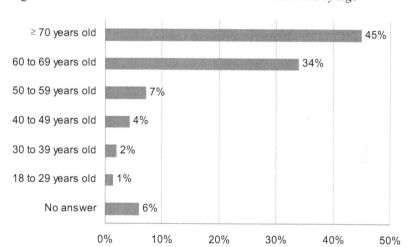

Source: See Techniker Krankenkasse (ed.) (2009), n = 6,187

Referring to one of the main purposes of the survey, the results showed that TK members with planned treatment in another EU member state share certain socio economic characteristics. This includes for example the age distribution. 79 per cent of the surveyed TK members who travel to other EU member states to receive planned treatment were 60 years and older.

Figure 4:   *TK Members with EU Cross-Border Treatments by Monthly Gross Income*

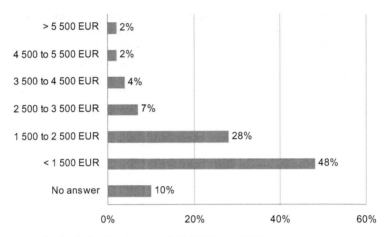

Source: See Techniker Krankenkasse (ed.) (2009), n = 5,572

Matching the results of the age distribution, 79 per cent of those members questioned were pensioners or retirees. An examination of the gross monthly income showed that it was mainly TK members on a lower income who received planned treatment in another EU member state.

These described results support the hypothesis that pensioners and retirees are the dominant and trend-setting target group with the highest patient mobility concerning EU cross-border treatment.

The picture is also complemented by the given answers concerning the most frequent underlying illnesses of patients with planned treatment. The illustration shows that more than two-thirds (70 per cent) suffer from diseases of their back or joints. Another 15 per cent had a cardiovascular disease and eight per cent suffered from a disease of their respiratory system.

Corresponding to the results of the patients' illnesses, the most popular types of treatment were remedies (55 per cent) and cure treatments (37 per cent). Regarding the four countries with the most planned EU cross-border treatment, Czech Republic, Poland, Italy and Hungary, the utilisation of remedies and spa treatments were even above-average.

Another hypothesis, which seems to be supported by the survey, was that the use of planned treatment in other EU member states is greater among those in the former West (65–84 per cent) than in the former East Germany (33–48 per cent). A possible reason for this could be the geographical proximity to the

122

traditional Eastern European spa resorts and the historical link between the former German Democratic Republic and Eastern-bloc countries. Further analyses have shown that a higher than average number of TK members from the former East Germany travel to the Czech Republic (29–40 per cent) and Poland (31–45 per cent) in order to receive medical treatment. By contrast, the use of such treatment by TK members from the former West Germany in the Czech Republic (11–25 per cent) and Poland (0–18 per cent) is much lower. The demand for receiving medical treatment in Hungary, however, is comparable in the former West Germany (8–22 per cent) and the former East Germany (7–17 per cent).

Figure 5:   *TK Members with EU Cross-Border Treatments by Illnesses*

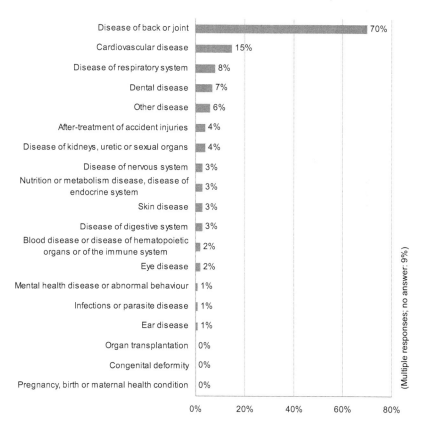

Source: See Techniker Krankenkasse (ed.) (2009), n = 8,219

A major difference to the EU cross-border survey 2008 and 2009 is that in 2010 TK's Scientific Institute for Benefit and Efficiency in Health Care WINEG (Wissenschaftliches Institut der TK für Nutzen und Effizienz im Gesundheitswesen) surveyed insurants – i.e. including dependent co-insurant – instead of paying independent members only.

Thus in the first survey part we contacted insurants concerning their experience who have already been in other EU member states for cross-border treatment. The underlying question was: Which experiences have TK insurants had with planned EU cross-border treatments in terms of quality, service and satisfaction? In this context WINEG is looking at the following three main areas of interest:

1. quality of the consultation and the service in the context of EU cross-border care provided by TK
2. information needs of the insurants and other factors influencing the decision to strive for EU cross-border treatment
3. satisfaction with the quality of the EU cross-border treatments and the service provided by doctors, hospitals and cure resorts.

In the second survey we selected for the first time a group of insurants who have no experience with EU cross-border care (yet) to ask them about their attitude, expectations and future behaviour in this field. The underlying question was: How will the demand for EU cross-border treatments by TK insurants develop in future?

The two questionnaires with respectively 42 and 30 questions were developed in summer 2010 and sent out to 50,000 insurants in November: 40,000 insurants with EU cross-border treatments in 2009 and 10,000 without. The responses were collected for eight weeks until January 2011. Based on the experience with response rates among TK insurants of former surveys concerning other topics, the response rates were again quite high, 33 per cent among insurants with experience and 27 per cent among insurants without. The following first results thus concerns a quality controlled data base of 16,023 insurants. As in the former survey of 2009 the insurants were mainly retirees aged 60 years and over with smaller incomes, i.e. less than 1,500 Euro. 24 per cent have an income less than 750 Euro.

---

12   The 2010 analysis of the results is still in progress. The publication in Wineg Wissen will follow soon.

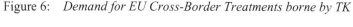

Figure 6: *Demand for EU Cross-Border Treatments borne by TK*

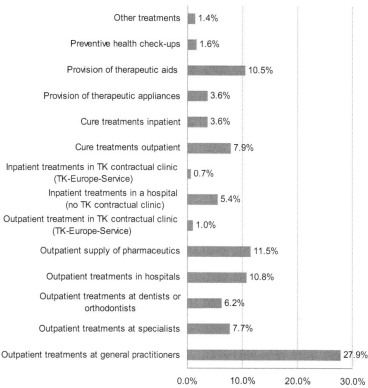

Source: TK Europe Survey 2010 (publication in progress), n = 14,728

The insurants had 12,251 EU cross-border treatments in total of which 39 per cent were planned and 61 per cent were unplanned, i.e. acute and emergency cases. Compared to the former survey the number of unplanned treatments has slightly increased and the number of planned treatments decreased.

The most popular EU member states as in the past are the Czech Republic, Poland, Italy and Hungary. Again these are mainly Eastern European countries except for the most favourite holiday destinations of the Germans, i.e. Italy.

Most of the EU cross-border treatments borne by TK are outpatient treatments in surgeries of general practitioners (31 per cent), followed by pharmaceuticals (13 per cent), outpatient treatments in hospitals (12 per cent) and remedies such as massages and inhalations (12 per cent). The second most important group of treatments demanded comprises cures (9 per cent), treatments in specialist surgeries or ambulatories (8 per cent), dentist and orthodontist treatments (7 per cent) as well as inpatient treatments in hospitals (6 per cent). The GP treatments and the inpatient treatments are the only ones to have increased as compared to the former survey.

The two main reasons for going abroad to get medical care have both been confirmed again: 26 per cent stated that cost savings were their most important motivation and 25 per cent thought that it was the combination of the treatment with a holiday trip. For nearly 80 per cent, the cost of the treatment(s) amounted to less than 1,000 Euro. Concerning the financing of these costs 66 per cent stated that they had to bear up to 500 Euro and 20 per cent between 500 Euro and 1,000 Euro.

Figure 7: *Costs of Treatment borne by the Insurants*

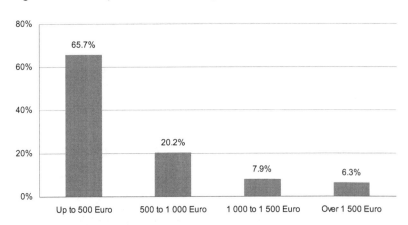

Source: TK Europe Survey 2010 (publication in progress), n = 2,856

Accordingly the majority of the surveyed insurants informed themselves about costs, i.e. the cost-sharing between them and TK and the possibilities to save costs. In addition to this the second area of major interest was quality, i.e. the medical quality and the quality of the facility's equipment.

Interestingly more than 78 per cent communicated with their doctor in German. Probably also as a consequence of this, 61 per cent of the insurants were very satisfied with the medical quality, i.e. the particularly result of their EU cross-border treatment, but also with the thoroughness of the examination, the medical consultation by the physicians and the qualification of all medical

126

Figure 8: *Needs for Information of Insurants concerning EU Cross-Border Care*

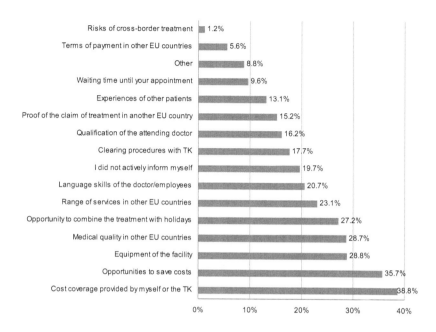

Source: TK Europe Survey 2010 (publication in progress), n = 13,287

staff in general. Moreover, they were also very satisfied with the organisation of the processes and the hygienic conditions in the surgeries, hospital and cure resorts, but also with possibilities to combine the treatment with a holiday trip, and the waiting times.

Figure 9: *Satisfaction with EU Cross-Border Treatments and Providers and TK*

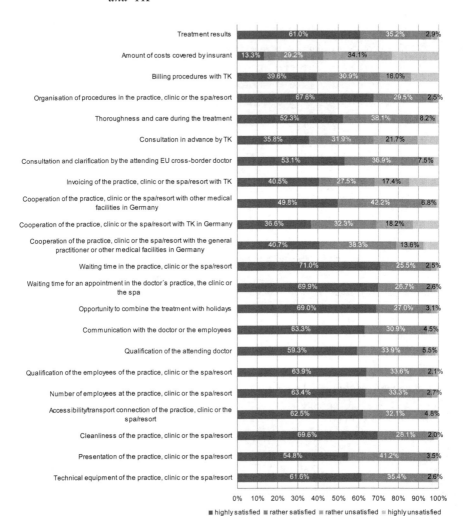

Source: TK Europe Survey 2010 (publication in progress), n = between 881 and 3,886 (varying according to the 22 different response categories)

In summary, at this early point of evaluation of the responses there are two first results to be observed concerning the main areas of interest we looked at:
1. The insurants who experienced EU cross-border treatments are extremely satisfied with the quality and service provided by doctors, hospitals and cure resorts.
2. The information need of these insurants, though, is focused on financing and cost aspects rather than quality aspects.

WINEG is currently evaluating the results of the two surveys in depth. A detailed report and further publications are in progress.

References

European Court of Justice (1998): Internet: http://europa.eu/index_de.htm, C-158/96 and C-120/95 (Kohl / Decker), rulings of 28 April 1998.
European Court of Justice (2001): Internet: http://europa.eu/index_de.htm, C-157/99 (»Smits / Peerbooms«), ruling of 12 July 2001.
European Court of Justice (2003): Internet: http://europa.eu/index_de.htm, C-385/99 (»Müller-Fauré / van Riet«), ruling of 13 May 2003.
European Court of Justice (2006): Internet: http://europa.eu/index_de.htm, C-372/04 (»Watts«) ruling of 16 May 2006 and 15 June 2006.
Klusen, Norbert (2008): in TK Analysis of EU Cross-Border Healthcare in 2007, Hamburg.
See European Commission / The Gallup Organization (2007). Cross-border health services in the EU – Analytical report, in: Flash Eurobarometer, No. 210.
Techniker Krankenkasse (ed.) (2003): Medizin und Europa, Ergebnisse der TK-Mitglieder-Befragung 2003, Hamburg.
Techniker Krankenkasse (ed.) (2009): German Patients en route to Europe, Hamburg. (TK EU Cross-Border Survey 2009, available at www.wineg.de)
Techniker Krankenkasse (ed.) (2008): TK Analysis of EU Cross-Border Healthcare in 2007, Hamburg. (TK Cross-Border Survey 2007, available at www.wineg.de)
Wagner C., Linder R. The Demand for EU Cross-Border Care: An Empirical Analysis. Journal of Management in Health Care 2010; 2(3).

Soziale Zukunft und Eurokrise – Selbstverwaltung, Staatsferne und höhere Freiheitsgrade als Markenzeichen des deutschen Systems in Zeiten politischer Anspannung

Günter Danner

Abstract

Our worlds of social security within the EU and beyond its borders are presently challenged to the extreme. A crisis scenario is striking at the core of the ability of the states to act when trying to master mounting debts, both public and private, as well as balancing socio-economically feasible policies with supra-national economic umbrellas of protection. In fact state bankruptcy of an EU member state will not be far away. Consequently mechanisms for worst-case scenarios of that ilk will have to be conceived before long. As a »second-rate« responsibility, the state remains the number one actor and financier in social systems of health care. In many other such fields – e.g. education and public infrastructure – signs of weakness and neglect are already there to be seen. Contrary to the situation in many other EU member states, the German health care system has remained relatively aloof from direct state influence. The reason for this is the tradition of self-administration, e.g. elected representatives of cost-carriers, as well as socially productive competition among such financing and purchasing institutions. As a matter of fact, the pillars of the German system's different structures are the above mentioned self-administration, competition among health funds and thus considerably more choice for patients. In this, the German model is almost unique in Europe. Even if too many hastily computed reform-bills have affected this model in a negative way, the basic substance is still to be rated among the most generous and »free«, if looked at from the point of view of the patient.

Subsidiarity and the right to decide upon the future of a national model at the national political level have been menaced by various forms of EU intervention, more often than not based on interpretations of the Single Market or the will of the EU Commission to co-influence the voluminous markets of health care within the framework of general EU deregulation. Preserving core qualities of the own system in order not to end up in a blurred world of theoretically proven standardised EU systems of health care out of touch with the local traditions and demands, is an important task today. This is all the more true since one should try to retain the national structures and capacities of a system which has met with public acceptance for decades. Thus cross-border exchange of ideas and experience has always been welcomed in Germany. There are in fact many highly interesting common problems and questions shared across borders and differences in system structure. The empowerment of actors at national or regional level to partake in such forms of co-opera-tion is thus ranking high on the agenda of the Techniker Krankenkasse, which in international and many other terms, has been ahead of the crowd for a long time.

Today's problems with public finances will pose enormous problems to gov-ernments the world over. As a rule of thumb it may be said that money can only be spent once – be this yet another protective umbrella for a weak EU member state, another bail-out of a bank, the education of our young or inno-vative investments in the future of health care. Seen from the German point of view, more self-administration will simply make it easier to guarantee that the known standard of care will not be subjected to political preferences of the moment. The Social Election – the vote for the representatives in the financing bodies of health care and pensions – to name just these – is on the agenda in Germany for this year. Its result is and will remain the cornerstone of the Ger-man social model. Many rightly believe in the growing importance of trans-border exchange, international comparison of solutions. Many Europeans, however, are already experiencing the inbuilt weaknesses of too much state influence in times of economic constraints. Lengthy waiting lists, linear rationing, under-funding of public services of general interest are all symp-toms of the ongoing – and by no means overcome – debt crisis. Not too many years ago, the German economic model with strong social responsibility used to be criticised for not being flexible enough, not sufficiently open toward the then new worlds of »dot.com-economies« or financial speculation on a grand scale. Some have even called it a »rust belt« of social policies then openly challenged. Nowadays – contrary to many international expectations – the German model of social consensus, productivity and technical innovation is evidently showing strength. Without the shrewd balance of innovation, pro-ductivity and social inclusion, this would not have been possible. In the world of health care, German institutions may benefit from ongoing EU activities to open up foreign providers to patients financed by social systems. The new Directive in its present final form will no longer endanger national legal structures and open up a bizarre »market« of atomised purchase of care based on pre-paid vouchers as was the wish of some in the European Parlia-ment. Instead much will depend on subtle bi- and multi-national agreements in order to guarantee statutory rights without endangering the respective national systems. More exchange and deeper co-operation will thus be more important tomorrow than they are today.

Zusammenfassung

Die Sozialwelten der EU-Mitgliedstaaten stehen vor bislang nicht gekannten Herausforderungen. Ein währungs- und wirtschaftspolitisches Krisenszenario bindet politische Kräfte und Haushaltsmittel. Schon zeigen erste »Gesundheitsreformen« in vielen Staaten die Handschrift der Krisenpolitik. Paniksparen, einseitige Belastungen und finanziell unerfüllbare Staatskompetenz mit qualitativem Niedergang bestimmen das Bild. Neben Deutschland kennen nur das sozialrechtlich völlig anders strukturierte Belgien und die Niederlande ein wettbewerbliches Miteinander von Kostenträgern im Gesundheitswesen. Bei uns wird dies durch Selbstverwaltung, Staatsferne und relativ höhere Freiheitsgrade für alle Systembeteiligten geprägt. Zugleich stehen als Ergebnis eines verstärkten internationalen Systemdialogs und einer intensivierten Suche nach den neusprachlich »Best Practice« benannten optimalen Lösungswegen viele technische Einzelheiten einander fremder Systemwelten im Fokus wissenschaftlicher Vergleiche. Dies wird zunehmen; vermutlich sind die Tage bis zu einem »Gesundheits-Pisa« nicht mehr fern. Wichtig ist es also, sich darüber klar zu werden, dass trotz der Nützlichkeit eines technischen Austauschs über die Systemgrenzen hinweg die fundamentalen Prinzipien der jeweiligen Sozialordnung in ihrer Bedeutung erkannt werden. Nur so ist ein Erhalt subsidiärer sozialrechtlicher Gestaltung – mithin des deutschen Sonderwegs – in Zeiten der offenen Methode der Koordinierung und anderer EU-Vergleichstechniken möglich.

Mehr EU-Vergemeinschaftung als Weg aus der Krise

Neue, bislang unbekannte Ansätze zur Vergemeinschaftung nationaler politischer Zuständigkeiten sind aus der Euro-Schuldenkrise erwachsen. Diese betreffen zunächst nicht direkt die nationale subsidiäre Sozialgesetzgebung. Allerdings ist ein mittelbarer Einfluss durch finanzielle Verpflichtungen der Regierungen im supranationalen Rahmen ebenso real wie die beschriebenen Sparaktivitäten in wichtigen öffentlichen Ausgabenbereichen. Zusätzlich zu den bedenklichen öffentlichen Schuldenlasten vor dem September 2008 traten enorme Verbindlichkeiten durch die Banken- und Finanzsystemsicherung auf. Im Rahmen der politischen Anstrengungen zum Erhalt der Marktrefinanzierungsfähigkeit verschiedener Euroländer wurden neue Verpflichtungen begründet. Dies geschah vermutlich einmal zur Aussendung eines Signals politischer Handlungsfähigkeit an die Märkte. Zum anderen kann unterstellt werden, dass das politische Unionsprojekt »EU« über kein Szenario für einen

Staatsbankrott verfügt. Möglicherweise ist dies ein technisches Erfordernis der unmittelbaren Zukunft, wenn es nicht mehr gelingt, von Zinstermin zu Zinstermin eines Wackelkandidatenstaates dessen wachsenden Geldbedarf zur Schuldenbedienung zu gewährleisten. Diese neue politische Situation trifft im Bereich des Gesundheitsschutzes auf ein bereits recht fortgeschrittenes Vergemeinschaftungsbemühen im Gesundheitsbereich. Dennoch ist die Systemvielfalt derzeit wohl nicht in akuter Gefahr. Auch nach Eröffnung neuer Horizonte in der Vergemeinschaftung und einer wachsenden Zahl »europäischer« Lösungsvorschläge für sozialökonomisch drängende Probleme wird sie im Sozialschutz Bestand haben. Zu unterschiedlich sind die jeweiligen nationalen Strukturen, als dass sie zu einem Einheitsmodell verschmelzen könnten. Zu ungeeignet wäre der augenblickliche Zeitpunkt für eine solche Idee. Die aktuelle Entwicklung deutet eher darauf hin, dass sich die Großzügigkeits- und Leistungsfähigkeitsunterschiede zwischen den einzelnen EU-Staaten fühlbar verschärfen werden. Aktuelle Formen des Staatsversagens – man denke an die verzweifelten Versuche der EU-Mitgliedstaaten, Staatsbankrotte in einer Reihe von Ländern zu verhindern – zeigen, in welche Richtung die Entwicklung geht. Die Harmonisierungsdiskussion der frühen 1990er Jahre ist somit aus systemtechnischer Sicht vermutlich erledigt. Strukturelle Anpassungsübungen aus funktionstechnischer Sicht könnten hingegen durchaus an Bedeutung gewinnen. Immerhin überlassen wir vor der Beschlussfassung den Haushaltsentwurf des Bundestages Brüsseler Stellen zur »Begutachtung«. Diese unausgesprochene partielle Preisgabe eines Souveränitätsrechtes kam im Zuge des händeringenden Suchens nach kollektiven Wegen aus den Haushaltskrisen bei uns nahezu unwidersprochen auf die politische Bühne. Verstetigt sie sich dort als mehr als ein vorübergehendes Krisenszenario, so könnte dies eine Wende in staatsunmittelbarer Souveränitätsausübung bedeuten. Nur infolge ihrer eindeutigen Staatsferne – ursächlich durch die Selbstverwaltung gewährleistet – vermag das deutsche GKV-System sich immerhin so lange in seiner gegenwärtigen Position zu behaupten, wie die finanztechnische Abhängigkeit vom noch verfügbaren staatlichen Steueraufkommen den Status quo nicht übersteigt. Gerät unsere Versorgungswelt in weitere Abhängigkeit von alljährlicher Zuweisung staatlicher Haushaltsmittel, die möglicherweise an anderer Stelle für die zahlreichen außerplanmäßigen EU-Rettungsschirme, »Bad Banks« oder ähnliche verpflichtende Konstrukte benötigt werden, so wird die Haushaltsplanung eines Kostenträgers problematisch. Das in vielen Staatssystemen, darunter auch dem britischen NHS oder den skandinavischen Volksheimen, praktizierte Mangelsteuerungsverfahren durch Wartelisten wäre mit dem sozialethischen Anspruch der deutschen GKV nicht vereinbar.

Wandel durch Annäherung in Zeiten der ökonomischen Ausnahmebedingungen?

Aus deutscher Sicht hätte eine strukturelle Annäherung die Preisgabe entscheidender Systemmerkmale zur Voraussetzung. Gerade weil Kernelemente des »deutschen Sonderwegs« in der Gesundheitsfinanzierung von denen in anderen Staaten abweichen und sich aus historischer Erfahrung die Mehrheit selten oder nie der Minderheit anzupassen pflegt, wäre eine solche Entwicklung für unser System verderblich. Neben den bereits national spürbaren schleichenden Ausweitungen der Staatszuständigkeit träte in diesem Fall ein Anpassungsdruck direkt von der »höheren« Ebene »Europa«. In Zeiten des europäischen Gesundheitsmarktes – seine Öffnung wurde durch die zur Jahresmitte 2011 in Kraft tretende EU-Richtlinie zu »Patientenrechten« in der grenzüberschreitenden Leistungsbeschaffung unlängst nachhaltig verdeutlicht – muss ein Systemweg mit hohen Alleinstellungsmerkmalen besondere EU-Kompetenz bereithalten. Staatsbewirkungsmodelle mit ihrem offiziösen Charakter sind dabei im Vorteil. Dennoch wird der mittelbare Druck des europäischen Vergemeinschaftungsgeschehens auf unsere GKV-Ordnung laufend stärker. Standen früher – in wirtschaftlich besseren Zeiten der EU als Raum – eher versorgungsorientierte Themen im Vordergrund des Interesses, so zeigt die Gegenwart ein Übergewicht von möglichst effizienten Rationierungsansätzen. In Zeiten knapper Mittel und teilweise drastisch eingeschränkter haushaltstechnischer Spielräume der öffentliche Hände stehen insbesondere solche Sozialleistungen auf dem Prüfstand, die Steuermittel erfordern. Entsprechend zeigt sich eine Tendenz, einseitig die Versicherten und besonders die kranken Versicherten zu belasten. In staatsfinanzierten Bewirkungsmodellen – etwa dem britischen Gesundheitsdienst, aber auch den eher sozialstaatsbereiteren skandinavischen Welten – zeigen sich unverhohlen Neigungen zum »bottlenecking«, d. h. zur indirekten oder direkten Vermeidung von Arzt-Patient-Kontakten, vorzugsweise in der öffentlich finanzierten Struktur. Dieser Umstand erklärt sich u. a. dadurch, dass die überwiegende Mehrzahl der EU-Systeme völlig oder vorwiegend aus Steuermitteln finanziert werden. Die Weltfinanzkrise hat jedoch mit dem Phänomen der Umwidmung der Folgen geplatzter Spekulationsblasen von der ursächlichen internationalen Finanzwirtschaft weg und in die öffentlichen Haushalte hinein neue Voraussetzungen geschaffen. Vermutlich auf Jahrzehnte sind die öffentlichen Hände in vielen Staaten mit kaum mehr vorstellbaren Schuldenlasten konfrontiert. Es liegt nahe, daraus einschneidende Veränderungen für alles abzuleiten, was traditionell staatliches Schuldenmachen politisch und volkswirtschaftlich gerechtfertigt hat. Infrastruktureller Niedergang, Panikprivatisierungen mit Nachhaltigkeitsverlusten im Versorgungszweck und lineare Kürzungen in allen staatlichen Ausgabenbereichen sind vielerorts bereits Realität. Dies gilt nicht etwa nur für solche Staaten, die bereits in der Risikozone eines Staatsbankrotts sind. Geradezu bedrohlich wird die aufgetürmte Schuldenmasse zudem dann, wenn inflationsbedingt die Zinsen fühlbar steigen sollten. Konsequenterweise sind staatsnahe oder staatsnah verwaltete Sozialversicherungssysteme, man denke an das durchaus leistungsfähige französische Bürgerversicherungsmodell, von diesen Entwicklungen auch dann bedroht, wenn die allgemeinen wirtschaftlichen Kerndaten sich zum Besseren wenden. Die Zweigleisigkeit aus vorhandenen bzw. seit 2008 aufgetürmten Verbindlichkeiten plus den Zukunftsbürgschaften im aktuellen oder bei weiteren Euro-Rettungsschirmen erhöhen somit den Druck auch auf solche Volkswirtschaften, deren gesunder produktivitätsbasierter Kern sich von den gerade ins Trudeln gekommenen Spekulationswelten vorteilhaft unterscheidet. Der »allgemeine« und mithin oft situativ-kurzfristige Sparzwang kann – insbesondere wenn politisch falsch gehandhabt – zu einer blinden Ausgabenblockade mit der Folge fehlender Zukunftsorientierung geraten. Dies wäre vermutlich für den sozialökonomischen Zusammenhalt und die wünschenswerte Nachhaltigkeit in der Haushaltspolitik ebenso gefährlich wie wahltaktische Klientelpolitik, die – in extremis – gerade Griechenland zum Verhängnis geworden ist. Die EU fordert und fördert zu Recht den Austausch nationaler Erfahrungen, auch und gerade mit dem Ziel der Eröffnung eines möglichst wechselseitigen Lernprozesses. Die Übernahme strukturfremder Details in die komplexe Ordnung eines sozialen Gesundheitssystems sollte jedoch streng nach einer Kompatibilitätsprüfung und keinesfalls unter dem ersten Eindruck systemfremder Beobachter erfolgen. Aus Sicht der Versicherten steht bei uns – im Unterschied zu vielen anderen EU-Sozialwelten – vieles auf dem Spiel. Passen wir uns systemtechnisch dabei in nicht sachgerechter Weise an andere Strukturen an, so kann es rasch zu einem Dominoeffekt kommen. Der Verzicht auf Selbstverwaltung bzw. deren Reduktion auf ornamentale Aufgaben nach Art des französischen Modells von 1997 hat zwar den Staat in eine mächtigere Position gebracht, jedoch weder die Zukunftsfestigkeit noch etwa die Verschuldungslage des Systems selbst verbessert. Wiederholt zeigte sich, dass nunmehr dem Staat unmittelbar zugewachsene Aufgaben entweder gar nicht oder in einer Weise erledigt wurden, die den unmittelbaren Erfordernissen der Systemsituation nicht entsprechen. Auffällig oft kam es zu wahltaktischen Kompromissen, an deren Ende gelegentlich mehr Probleme der Lösung harrten als weniger. Der gegenwärtige spontane Drang zur Einsparung um jeden Preis dürfte sich in diesem Zusammenhang kaum positiv auswirken.

Haushaltskonsolidierung, Euro-Rettungspakete und politischer Stellenwert des Gesundheitsschutzes

Die Haushaltskonsolidierung hat einen bedeutenden Stellenwert, Sozialschutz und Bildungspolitik als Produktivitätsträger der Zukunft allerdings auch. Die Volkswirtschaften der EU haben in der Krisenzeit deutlich gemacht, was nachhaltig zählt: Die einst als »celtic tiger« überbewertete irische Spekulationslandschaft ist vermutlich für immer dahin; die früher als »sozialparadiesisch-ideenlose Rostzone« verhöhnte deutsche exportorientierte Produktionswirtschaft zeigt momentan Wachstumswerte wie seit vielen Jahren nicht mehr. Eine Problemkombination »Euro-Staatsverschuldung« und der politische Umgang mit der Gemeinschaftswährung bindet enorme politische Kräfte. Unklar ist, ob die politischen Anstrengungen auf Bewahrung des großen EU-Modells eines anzustrebenden Superstaates ausgerichtet sind – hier wäre US-artig zu handeln – oder ob proportional zum Verflechtungsgrad durchaus nationalstaatlich individuelle Verantwortlichkeiten erhalten bleiben sollen, mit allen denkbaren Konsequenzen. Pointierter ausgedrückt steht zur Debatte, ob der Euro als Zahlungsmittel – dies benutzen auch Bankrotteure – oder als Klammer des beschriebenen Superstaatsmodells »gerettet« werden soll. Unklar ist ferner, weshalb der Euro nachhaltig geschädigt würde, wenn eines oder auch zwei seiner volkswirtschaftlich auf eigene Rechnung handelnden Mitgliedstaaten insolvent würden. Dieser formulierte Nichthaftungsgrundsatz war immerhin der deutsch geprägte Geist des Maastrichter Vertrages, den wir mit der augenblicklichen EU-Politik partiell verlassen haben. Die nahe Zukunft wird zeigen, wie lange die Rettungsschirmpolitik tatsächlich tragen kann. Gäbe es dabei keine Grenzen – auch solche, die noch einer Definition harren –, so steht am Ende wohl eine strukturelle Identität, unabhängig vom nationalen Umgang mit volkswirtschaftlicher Primärlogik. Ob die weltweite Spekulation zudem durch die Garantieversprechen nicht möglicherweise mehr angeheizt wird als durch einzelne Staatsbankrotte, das ist Auffassungssache. Fakt ist jedenfalls, dass Staatstitel von Wackelstaaten kurzfristiges Renditepotential haben. Ist dies nun »mehr Spekulation« oder die Lösung des eigentlichen Problems? Wie entscheidungsrelevant ist schließlich die Summe der Staatsbonds von Schwachstaaten in deutschen oder anderen institutionellen Anlageportfolios? Möglicherweise »retten« wir uns am Ende aufwändig selbst vor unüberschaubarem Abschreibebedarf. Was geschieht allerdings, wenn das gegenwärtige Verfahren nicht mehr greift? In jedem Fall steht eine isolierte nationale Stabilitätspolitik dann nach Erschöpfung der Transferfähigkeit einer Volkswirtschaft strenggenommen auf der Verliererseite. Immerhin ist auch die Stützungskraft des Stärksten endlich, wenn er am Ende allein steht. Wird diese Grenze bald – auch unter europapolitischen »Schmerzen« – festgelegt, so ist ein solches Schicksal möglicherweise abwendbar.

Die Krise unterstreicht, dass es auch in der Eurozone keine Strukturidentität der Mitgliedstaaten mit beliebigem Vonsichweisen der Verantwortung für eigenes vergangenes politisches und ökonomisches Handeln geben kann. Problematisch bleibt der so genannte »fallout«. Wie viel politische und demokratiestabilisierende sozialökonomische Substanz kann an welchem Ort und zulasten welcher Personenkreise abgebaut werden, bevor der Schaden irreparabel ist und die Demokratie zu leiden beginnt. Gerade das einstige nationale Konsensmodell der Niederlande zeigt in jüngster Vergangenheit eine viele überraschende Tendenz zur Gewichtung monothematischer Parteien mit der Folge, dass es diesen gelang, andere zum Regieren in teilweise politischer Abhängigkeit zu verführen. Je nach nationaler Gewohnheit dürfte die Schmerzschwelle da unterschiedlich sein. Deutschlands großzügige Sozialwelt zeigt vermutlich geringe Tendenzen zum supranationalen solidarischen Verzicht. Dieser wäre auch mit dem Beitragsfinanzierungsprinzip kaum vereinbar, da solcher Art bewirkte Mittel wesentlich zielbestimmter auszugeben sind als die nach jährlicher Haushaltsberatung neu verteilungsfähigen Steuermittel des Staates. Jeder potentiellen EU-Transferunion im Gesundheitsschutzbereich sind damit äußerst enge Grenzen gesetzt.

Teilhabegebot und sozialer Gesundheitsschutz in Krisenzeiten

Eine Versorgungswelt im Gesundheitswesen darf kein Schönwettermodell sein. Gerade die Gegenwart erfordert besondere Anstrengungen, das hohe Schutzniveau zu erhalten. Deutschland durchlebt eine ökonomisch zufriedenstellende Wachstumsphase. Produktivität, Innovationsvermögen und Absatzmöglichkeiten, insbesondere in den globalen Wachstumszentren Asiens und Lateinamerikas, stehen dafür ebenso wie die Solidität deutscher Betriebe – klein und groß – und der vergleichsweise große soziale Zusammenhang unserer Gesellschaft.

Nicht zuletzt aus diesem Grund muss der sozialökonomischen Betrachtung Raum gegeben werden. Das traditionelle Europa der nationalen sozialökonomischen Horizonte und Rechtswelten ächzt unter nicht voraussehbaren exogenen Belastungen. In den Leidensstaaten der Bankrottnähe greift die Politik unmittelbar in die soziale Realität ein. In anderen Ländern – so auch bei uns – drohen in der abstrakten Dominanz der auf Kostenreduktion fixierten Haushaltspolitik über der sozialökonomischen Gesamtverantwortung durchaus bereits bedenkliche Langfristfolgen. Staatsferne – ohne Selbstverwaltung nicht zu gewährleisten – garantiert einen nach wie vor hinreichenden Spielraum der unmittelbar betroffenen Akteure, den man ausbauen sollte, statt ihn einzuengen. Die relativ höheren Freiheitsgrade in unserem System ermöglichen ein wettbewerbliches Nebeneinander von Kostenträgern mit entspre-

138

chender Einstellung zum Versicherten ebenso wie eine sich von den staatlich vereinheitlichten Bewirkungsmodellen unterscheidende Angebotsstruktur. Wo eine freie Arztwahl – auch des Facharztes in der ambulanten Versorgung – nicht mehr möglich ist, ist der Schritt zur systemtechnischen Patientenlenkung ohne nennenswerte Berücksichtigung der individuellen Präferenzen rasch vollzogen. Dieses Privileg genießen im EU-Systemumfeld nur wenige Staaten ohne legale oder illegale Direktvergütung durch den Kranken. Auch bei uns könnten die Wettbewerbselemente im Interesse eines Gewinns an Vernunftlösungen im Allokationsprozess durchaus ausgeweitet werden. Fehlte der Politik dazu in der Vergangenheit der Mut oder der Wille – viele gehen erstaunlicherweise nach wie vor davon aus, dass nur der Staat »wirklich gerecht« verteilen könne –, so mag die Krise mit ihrer Schwächung des staatlichen Handlungsvermögens hier ein Umdenken anstoßen. Die Suche nach bestmöglichen Lösungswegen dürfte sich von plumper Verstaatlichung oder blindem Markt- und Privatisierungsglauben nahezu gleich weit entfernt haben. Immerhin hat das eklatante Marktversagen der internationalen Finanzwelt zusammen mit der Delegation der Folgen und Verbindlichkeiten an die Regierungen zum Istzustand der Krise beigetragen. Zwar vertritt die Bundesregierung in der EU durchaus härtere Positionen im Umgang mit den Krisenverantwortlichen, doch ist in Brüssel stets nur ein gemeinsamer Nenner politisch zu verwirklichen. Als Fazit darf festgehalten werden, dass der nationale Verantwortlichkeitsrahmen – allen Vergemeinschaftungswünschen und -tendenzen zum Trotz – nicht ausgedient hat.

Sozialer Gesundheitsschutz und staatsferner Handlungsspielraum

In der eigentlich erforderlichen gesundheitspolitischen Diskussion ginge es um mittel- und langfristige Versorgungsszenarien mit Anbindung an Demografie und Morbiditätsprognosen. Sie wäre nur parteienübergreifend zu führen, weil der Zeithorizont leicht eine Legislaturperiode übersteigt. Für die Zukunftsfähigkeit unseres Systems ist sie unerlässlich. Nur so haben auch künftige Generationen vielleicht die Hoffnung auf ein befriedigendes Gesundheitsmodell in vergleichsweise höherer Leistungsbereitschaft, Berechenbarkeit und Versichertenmitgestaltung. Eine solche Konditionierung des Systems ist zudem – wo wäre dies relevanter als in einer Veröffentlichung aus dem Umkreis der Techniker Krankenkasse – unabdingbare Voraussetzung für eine künftige Angebots- und Systemvielfalt auf Seiten der Kostenträger. Verschwindet die Selbstverwaltung, so tritt zwingend »mehr Staat« an ihre Stelle. Sozialverträglicher Wettbewerb – Voraussetzung für zukunftsweisenden Kreativitätsgehalt in der Führung eines Dienstleistungsunternehmens sozialpolitischer Aufgabenstellung – wäre hinfort weniger relevant als die ultrakurzfristige Einhaltung kleinteilig formulierter und schon einmal sachfremder Politikvorgaben. Manch ein »Reformgesetz« bekommt politisch erst gar nicht die Zeit für eine Systemeinwirkung. Da bleiben oft nur Kostendämpfungsgesetzgebung der kurzatmigen Art und Reform der Reformen übrig. »Mehr Staat« in der heutigen Zeit wäre gefährlich. Statt freiheitsorientierter Aufgabenbewältigung in größtmöglicher Nähe zu den Betroffenen in ihren Solidargemeinschaften – ein prozesstechnisches Schlüsselelement im deutschen Sozialschutz der GKV – würde eingeebnet bis zur Nulllinie. Die Wertfiktion politischer »Gleichheit« – auch im Weniger oder Nichts – würde dann eine zugegebenermaßen anstrengendere laufende schöpferische Bewältigung sozialwirtschaftlicher Managementaufgaben als Zielvorgabe ersetzen. Leidtragende wären unmittelbar die Kranken und die gesunden Versicherten, mittelbar auch der nationale Gesundheitsmarkt mit immerhin über 4,2 Millionen Arbeitsplätzen. Bewahren wir hingegen aktiv die Kernelemente unseres deutschen Sonderwegs, bauten wir Selbstverwaltung tatsächlich und mit dem erforderlichen politischen Mut aus, so wäre die Chance gegeben, sich systemtechnisch den vielen Risiken zu entziehen und Vielfalt, Optionen, Wahlmöglichkeiten und Mitwirkung in sozialverantwortlicher Wettbewerblichkeit an kommende Generationen weiterzureichen.

Wer vertritt die Versicherteninteressen?

Der umfassende Versorgungsanspruch eines Staatsmodells – etwa des NHS – regelt sich auf nationaler Ebene bzw. in Großbritannien durch die jeweils für die Landesteile zuständigen Verwaltungsbehörden. Dies ist ein eindeutiger »Top-down«-Prozess, bei dem die Basismitwirkung nachträglich aufgepfropft als regionale Erscheinung feststellbar ist. Künftige Strukturen des NHS schaffen gar einen Hauptakteur – die hausärztliche Versorgung – als allgemeinen Mittelverwalter, auch zum eigenen Nutzen. Die Abschaffung der Primary Care Trusts (PCT), die bislang regionale Mittelzuweisungen vorgenommen haben, soll den Dienst »entbürokratisieren«. Kritiker befürchten jedoch eine auch von betriebswirtschaftlichen Erwägungen getragene Mittellenkung durch die »GPs«, die weitgehend keine freiberuflichen Hausärzte mehr sind, sondern mehr und mehr Beschäftigte profitorientierter Dienstleistungskonzerne. Ob die Abwägungsaufgaben der ehemaligen PCT tatsächlich besser im Sinne der Patientennähe vorgenommen werden, wird die Zukunft zeigen. Immerhin forderte die heutige Mitregierungspartei der Liberaldemokraten noch im Wahlkampf an dieser Stelle die Einführung einer »Selbstverwaltung« in Gestalt von Vertretern der Patienten. Davon ist heute nicht mehr die Rede. Was als Patientenmitgestaltungsoption bleibt, ist nicht gewaltig. Wie an vielen Orten gibt es für bestimmte Patientenkollektive (Selbsthilfe-

oder Interessengruppen) kommunal organisierte Angebote, ähnlich wie in Frankreich, wo spezielle kommunale Brennpunktaktivitäten – allerdings vorzugsweise in sozialen Brennpunkten – in jüngerer Zeit geschaffen wurden. Mit der deutschen Selbstverwaltung sind solche weitgehend die Teilaspekte berührenden Einrichtungen nicht direkt vergleichbar. Weder können diese in das Geschäft des Kostenträgers – etwa den Mittelfluss – eingreifen oder dies auch nur mitbestimmen, noch sind in den meisten Fällen gesetzliche Kompetenzen definiert.

Es soll nicht bestritten werden, dass auch bei uns zu viel Staat in manchen Handlungsfeldern erkennbar wird. Von der herrschenden Realität im Ausland sind wir jedoch weit entfernt. Selbstverwaltung berührt in einem anderen Kontext bei uns auch das Leistungs- und Vertragsgeschehen. Wo in Großbritannien Verwaltungsbedienstete oder künftig »Konzessionäre« des NHS sowie Politiker und vom System beschäftigte Leistungserbringer »auf Weisung« tätig werden, tritt bei uns in der ambulanten Versorgung die individuelle Verantwortung des freiberuflich niedergelassenen Arztes und Facharztes. Dies ist, betriebswirtschaftlich betrachtet, eine mittelständische Lösung in freier Berufsausübung. Auf der Basis des vertragsgestützten Leistungseinkaufs durch unsere Krankenkassen ist somit die Sozialgebundenheit des Versorgungsvorganges weitgehend gewährleistet. Das ist in nahezu allen anderen EU-Staaten anders, wo entweder abhängig Beschäftigte die Versorgung ausführen bzw. das Kostenträgersystem vorhandene Strukturen in kommunaler oder anderer Trägerschaft nutzt. Wahlmöglichkeiten hat der Patient dort nur in den seltensten Fällen. Im internationalen Schrifttum findet sich gelegentlich Kritik am »komplizierten« und »intransparenten« deutschen Modell. Zugegebenermaßen ist die Bürokratie in der Versorgung – nicht immer ohne negative Auswirkungen auf das so wichtige Arzt-Patient-Verhältnis – in der jüngeren Vergangenheit stark gestiegen. Dies ist jedoch auch in den Staatsmodellen der Fall. Nicht von ungefähr möchte der NHS nach Jahren der Intensivierung der Verwaltung nun Abertausende von »Verwaltungsstellen« ersatzlos einsparen. Die allgemeine Entwicklung zur höchstmöglichen »Genauigkeit«, eine verbreitete wissenschaftliche Liebe zu Zahlen, Daten und Fakten – auch solchen, die u. U. nicht eben sehr prozessrelevant sind – gibt oft demjenigen Recht, der mehr und ausführlichere Datensammlungen aufweisen kann. Ob und in welchem Umfang sie für die Nachhaltigkeit der am Kranken erbrachten individuellen Leistung und deren sozialökonomische Fortschreibungsfähigkeit in die Zukunft unverzichtbar sind, darf bezweifelt werden. Die so immens wichtige zwischenmenschliche Dimension des »Heilens« wird durch sie kaum verbessert.

Auch nach Jahren einer, freundlich formuliert, überaus diskussionswürdigen Gesundheitspolitik kann unser System – bei allen Mängeln im Detail – viele Vorteile aufweisen. Diese gilt es zu bewahren. Den »Markencharakter« unserer Angebotsstrukturen gilt es zudem deutlich zu positionieren, auch im internationalen Umfeld. Agieren ist ebenso gefragt wie der Mut, zum nationalen Weg »Ja« zu sagen. Der Vergemeinschaftungsdruck aus Schuldenbergen und dem Streben nach immer mehr »europäischen« Lösungen birgt die Gefahr, dass es hier sonst zu strukturellen Anpassungen an den dann (noch) existierenden EU-Durchschnitt der Versorgungssysteme kommen könnte. Dies wäre sowohl für die nach deutschem Recht versicherten Personen nachteilig als auch gefährlich für die Breitenzustimmung zum europäischen Friedenswerk. Eine umsichtige nationale Politik – dies wird zunehmend und lagerübergreifend erkannt – wird der Entmachtung des Nationalstaates nicht mehr ohne weiteres folgen, wenn damit bisher selbstverständliche soziale Substanz zur Disposition abstrakter politischer Handlungsebenen steht. Nicht plumpe EU-Verweigerung, sondern beständige und belastbare Wahrung unveräußerbarer Interessen – auch und gerade im Sinne eines akzeptierten, nicht ertragenen Europäisierungsgrades – sollte dabei die Richtung vorgeben. In der unmittelbaren Organisation der Kostenträger der gesetzlichen Krankenversicherung sind daher Selbstverwaltung und der mit ihr eng verbundene Gedanke von struktureller Vielfalt, Mitgestaltung, Wahloptionen und sozialverträglichem Wettbewerb nach Möglichkeit auszubauen. Weniger Staat sollte nicht »mehr Markt« dorthin bringen, wo dieser möglicherweise die gestellten Aufgaben nicht befriedigend zu lösen vermag. Erst der durch Selbstverwaltung glaubhaft begründete Anspruch auf Sozialverträglichkeit macht aus einem effizient verwalteten Kostenträger einen Bestandteil der nationalen Sozialstaatskultur. Im Dialog mit dem Ausland sollten die Deutschen mehr Mut haben, eigene Lösungen, auch wenn diese kompliziert und schwieriger international vermittelbar zu sein scheinen, als probate Wege zu beschreiben, nicht notwendigerweise mit missionarischem Charakter, allerdings auch nicht mit der in der Vergangenheit feststellbaren Neigung zur positiven Überbewertung des Fremden an sich. Die einzelnen Elemente des deutschen Sonderweges kennen – gleich einem komplizierten Bausatz – eine ausgeprägte Interdependenz. So wird man die »Freiberuflichkeit« in der Leistungserbringerschaft nicht ohne Rückwirkungen auf den Anbietermarkt pauschal verändern. Wo ein individuelles Arzt-Patient-Verhältnis weitgehend als positiver Konsens angesehen wird, sind rasche Eingriffe in die strukturelle Substanz möglicherweise perspektivisch von Übel. Ein Muss in der künftigen Systemdiskussion ist der Abschied von weitgehend inhaltsleeren Debatten um Schlagwörter: Weder Kostenerstattung noch »Steuerfinanzierung« oder »Privatisierung« sind hinreichende Bestimmungsgrößen für eine systemtechnische Zukunftsfähigkeit. Die Beweislast, tatsächlich besser zu sein als die traditionelle Lösung, liegt auch künftig beim Neuen. Radikalreformen verbieten sich angesichts der allgemeinen sozialökonomischen Probleme von selbst. Es gilt hingegen, im permanenten Dialog der Betroffenen über Lagergrenzen hinweg Schnittmengen bei strukturellen Gemeinsamkeiten auszuloten, die seitens der Akteure einer mehr und mehr von »übergeordneten« Dingen belasteten Politik thematisch nähergebracht werden müssen. Die »Interessenpartei« von einst – kaum an der Macht, so sind alle »meine« kühnsten Wünsche Wirklichkeit – hat ausgedient. Schon heute sind die Lösungsvorschläge der Parteien – um Rhetorik entkleidet – kaum verschieden. Im Gesundheitswesen werden nur zu oft uralte Requisiten und Worthülsen als Ersatz für Lösungsvorschläge bemüht. Die Mühe einer Neuorientierung wird sich jedoch lohnen: Im EU-Umfeld kann das deutsche Gesundheitssystem durchaus positiv abstrahlen, Alternativen und Angebote vorhalten sowie deutlich machen, dass es in seinem Anderssein nicht zur Disposition steht. Es kann auch europäischen Mehrwert leisten, sowohl durch vorbildliches »Patient empowerment« als auch durch leistungsfähige Strukturen, die für Ausländer offen sind, ohne Inländer zu benachteiligen. Schaffen wir dazu die Möglichkeiten im grenzüberschreitenden Dialog und bei uns daheim. Die Zeit ist reif!

Authors

Dr Jens Christian Baas, born in 1967, is Member of the Board of Management of Techniker Krankenkasse (TK), a leading German health insurance company and a non-profit organisation. He studied medicine at the University of Heidelberg and the University of Minnesota (US). After his graduation he worked in the university hospitals of Heidelberg and Munster, focusing on transplant surgery. In 1999, Dr Baas moved to the Boston Consulting Group. From 2007 to 2010, he was Partner, Managing Director and European Leader of BCG's Payers and Providers practice. In his work with leading European payer organisations he focused on the optimization of patient care, e.g. by developing and implementing DMP and quality control systems. In 2011 he became Member of the Board of TK.

Dr Martin Bardsley is Head of Research. Martin is an experienced heath service analyst and researcher. Before joining The Nuffield Trust he worked for the Healthcare Commission leading a team developing and implementing approaches to the use of information for risk-based regulation. This work impacted on a number of areas of work across the Commission including the assessment of core standards, topic-based reviews and in support of investigations. He was also one of the key architects of the Annual Health Check that emerged in 2005 as a replacement for star ratings. Martin also spent three years at CHI as an Assistant Director in Research and Information where he helped shape the approach to analysis of qualitative information. Prior to working as a regulator, Martin led the Health of Londoners Project – a public information group working for all London's health authorities and a precursor to the London Health Observatory. Over a period of six years, the project produced a variety of reports and analyses of health in the capital – including the first public health report for Greater London. Previously he worked at CASPE research (a DH-funded health services research group) where his special interests were in outcome measurement and case mix classification. He was one of the original researchers using DRGs in the UK.

Sebastian Bauhoff is a Postdoctoral Fellow in the Department of Health Policy at Harvard Medical School. His research is at the intersection of health economics, applied microeconomics and empirical methods. Dr Bauhoff holds a PhD in Health Policy (Economics track) from Harvard University and a MPA in International Development from the Harvard Kennedy School.

Biggi Bender, spokesperson on health care policy, was born 1956 in Düsseldorf and started her political career 1984 as legal advisor, later policy expert on women´s issues, for the Green Party in the provincial legislature of Baden-Württemberg. She was elected to the provincial legislature as member for Stuttgart inner-city constituency in 1988. After that she was the leader of the Greens in the provincial legislature. From 1992 until 2000 Biggi was deputy leader of the Greens in the provincial legislature and chairperson of the Committee on Women, Family, Further Education and Art until 1996. She has been a longstanding member of national party councils, e.g. Länder, women, and of the executive committee of the Greens in Baden-Württemberg since 1999. Biggi has been deputy chairperson of the Baden-Württemberg branch of the DPWV (Paritätischer Wohlfahrtsverbund – German Federation of Charitable Organisations) since 2001. She was elected to the 15th Bundestag for the constituency of Stuttgart II in 2002 and re-elected 2005 and 2009. Biggi Bender is also a member of the committee on Health and an alternate member of the committee on Labour and Social Affairs.

Prof. Reinhard Busse, Dr med. MPH FFPH, is department head for health care management in the Faculty of Economics and Management at Technische Universität Berlin, Germany. He is also a faculty member of Charité, Berlin's medical faculty as well as Associate Head of Research Policy and Head of the Berlin hub of the European Observatory on Health Systems and Policies, a member of several scientific advisory boards as well as a regular consultant for WHO, the EU Commission, the Worldbank, OECD and other international organisations within Europe and beyond as well as national health and research institutions. He is the director of the annual Observatory's summer schools in Venice and the coordinator of the EU-funded project »EuroDRG: Diagnosis-Related Groups in Europe: towards Efficiency and Quality« (7th Framework; 2009–2011).

Anita Charlesworth is Chief Economist. Before joining the Nuffield Trust as Chief Economist in September 2010, Anita had been Chief Analyst and Chief Scientific Advisor at the Department of Culture, Media and Sport since 2007. Previously, Anita was Director of Public Spending at the Treasury, where she led the team working with Sir Derek Wanless on his reform for NHS funding in 2002. Anita has a Masters in Health Economics from York University and has worked as an Economic Advisor in the Department of Health and for Smithkline Beecham pharmaceuticals in the UK and US. Anita is vice-chair of NHS Islington, a trustee of Tommy's baby charity, member of the EPSRC Societal Issues Panel and member of the British Academy Centre for Policy Advisory Board.

Dr Zack Cooper is an Economic and Social Research Council Post Doctoral Fellow in Economics at the Centre for Economic Performance at the London School of Economics. He did his undergraduate work at the University of Chicago and his Masters and PhD at the London School of Economics. Zack's work focuses on the impact of competition in hospital and insurance markets, incentive structure and payment system design. More broadly, he is interested in using market forces to create effective incentives within the public sector. His most recent work looking at the impact of hospital competition in the English National Health Service is forthcoming in the Economic Journal. In addition to his academic work, Zack has worked as an advisor and speech-writer to several policy makers and politicians. Zack appears frequently in the popular press, including on the BBC, Sky News, ABC, CBS and National Public Radio. Zack's research has been cited in the Financial Times, the Times, the Independent, the Washington Post, the Evening Standard, the Economist, the Health Service Journal and the Guardian and he is a regular contributor to the Huffington Post.

Günter Danner, M.A., PhD, born 1955, German and British national. University studies of history, economics and international relations in the UK, Germany, the US and South Africa. Since 1982 working for the Techniker Krankenkasse in Hamburg as a press spokesperson and later as an analyst of political and socio-economic affairs in Germany and abroad. Today working as the personal advisor to the CEO and the Board of Management of one of the largest German health funds with approx. eight million insured and 10,000 employees on socio-economic, political and international affairs. Since 1993, in addition to the abovementioned, working for the permanent Liaison Bureau of German Social Security institutions in Brussels, since 1997 as the Deputy Director of this institution. Since 1992 as an international expert on health care systems, their administration, performance and guiding political background, frequent assignments on Commission projects in Central and East-European Countries (CEEC) undergoing social and economic transition as well as Russia and China. Numerous publications on issues dealing with international comparison of social protection, in particular health care. Author of the book »Die Europäische Union am Scheideweg Wohlstandsprojekt, Wettlaufgesellschaft oder Wolkenkuckucksheim«, Meusch Verlag, Hamburg 2004. Frequent invitations as a speaker at national and international conferences on health and EU-related matters. Regular academic teaching commitments e.g. in France, Germany, Sweden and the US.

Prof. Dr med. Jörg F. Debatin, born in 1961 in Bonn, German. Jörg F. Debatin studied medicine at the Medical School of the University of Heidelberg where he graduated in 1987. He completed his Residency in Diagnostic

Radiology at Duke University Medical Center and subsequently moved to Stanford University Medical Center for Fellowship in Abdominal Imaging. As a Diplomate of the American Boards of Radiology he took up a position as Associate Professor of Radiology and Chief of Magnetic Resonance Imaging in July 1993 at Zürich University Hospital. Following an »Executive MBA« Training at the University of St. Gallen, Switzerland, he was Appointed Professor and Chairman of the Department of Diagnostic and Interventional Radiology at the University Hospital in Essen in August 1999. In November 2003 Jörg F. Debatin moved to the University Medical Center Hamburg-Eppendorf where he serves in the position of Medical Director and Chief Executive Officer. Since 2006 he has been member of the Board of Directors of the CDU Council of Economic Advisors.

Dr Jennifer Dixon, Director of The Nuffield Trust, has researched and written widely on health care reform in the UK and internationally. She trained originally in medicine, practising mainly paediatric medicine, before a career in policy analysis. She has a Masters in public health and a PhD in health services research from the London School of Hygiene and Tropical Medicine. Until January 2008 she was director of policy at the King's Fund, London. She was a Harkness Fellow in New York in 1990 studying the obstacles to comprehensive health reform in the US, and was the policy advisor to the Chief Executive of the National Health Service between 1998 and 2000. She is currently a board member of the Audit Commission, and until recently on the Board of the Healthcare Commission. She is visiting Professor at both LSE and at Imperial College. Recent specific research interests have been in developing risk stratification and risk adjustment techniques for application in the NHS, in particular in resource allocation and identifying high-risk patients for case management. She helped to design the evaluation of the DH funded 'whole system demonstrator' project, which is a large complex randomised controlled trial, and is leading a key theme – the impact of telecare and tele-health on service use and costs. In 2009 Jennifer was elected as a Fellow of the Royal College of Physicians.

Dipl.-Ing. Alexander Geissler has been research fellow and PhD candidate at the Department of Health Care Management at the Technical University Berlin since November 2008 where he studied Economics and Engineering with an emphasis on health economics, health care management and logistics. Currently, he is conducting research on incentives and payment methods for the financing of hospitals and their impact on the quality and efficiency of service delivery in the framework of the EuroDRG project.

Prof. Dr Norbert Klusen, born in 1947, is Chairman of the Board of Management of Techniker Krankenkasse (TK), a leading German health insurance company and a non-profit organisation. He studied Economics, Sociology, Psychology and Political Sciences at Technical University (RWTH) Aachen and Technical University (TU) Berlin and graduated in Business Management at TU Berlin where he also received his PhD in Economics (Dr rer. oec.). Prof. Klusen worked in the management of several international companies. He was Board Member and Human Resources Director of a joint-stock company in the machinery and vehicle construction sector until 1993 when he became Chief Operating Officer at Techniker Krankenkasse. Since 1996, he has been Chairman of the Board of Management at TK. Besides his duties at TK, he lectures International Health Care Policy and Systems as Professor at Leibniz University Hanover. He has also been Professor of Health Care Economics and Health Care Policy at the University of Applied Sciences of Western Saxony since 1998 and visiting Professor of Health Management and Health Policy at University of Michigan, Ann Arbor (2009).

Dr Alistair McGuire is Professor in Health Economics at LSE Health and Social Care, based at the London School of Economics. Formerly, Dr McGuire was Professor in Health Economics at City University, London. Prior to this, he was a tutor in economics at Pembroke College, University of Oxford, and a research fellow at the Health Economics Research Unit, University of Aberdeen. Professor McGuire has 15 years' experience in the economics of health care, has written numerous books, articles, and reports on the topic, and consulted several pharmaceutical companies on economic evaluation. A former member of the UK Government's Cabinet Office Advisory Council on Science and Technology, he has also served on a number of research committees including the UK Medical Research Council Experts Committee, the MRC Steering Committee on the UK Prospective Diabetes Study, and the Economic and Social Science Research Committee on Food and Nutrition. He has served on a number of NUCE Committees and, additionally, has acted as a World Health Organization consultant, and has advised many international companies and reimbursement agencies.

Thomas G. McGuire, PhD, is a Professor of health economics in the Department of Health Care Policy at Harvard Medical School. His research focuses on the design and impact of health care payment systems, the economics of health care disparities, and the economics of mental health policy. Dr McGuire has contributed to the theory of physician, hospital, and health plan payment. Two jointly authored papers received »best paper of the year« awards for 2008, from Academy Health for work on physician-patient interaction and from the National Institute for Health Care Management for work on incentives in managed care plans. Also in 2008, he received the Everett Mendelsohn Excellence in Mentoring Award from Harvard's Graduate School of Arts and Sciences. He is a recipient of the Elizur Wright Award from the American Association of Risk and Insurance, the Arrow Award from the International Health Economics Association, and the Carl Taube Award from the American Public Health Association. Dr McGuire is a member of the Institute of Medicine, and a coeditor of the Journal of Health Economics. He received his BA degree from Princeton University and his PhD degree in economics from Yale University.

Anne-Katrin Meckel, born 1983, got her degree in business administration with the main focus on health management from the Friedrich-Alexander-University Erlangen-Nürnberg. She received the Unikosmos Marketing Award 2009/2010 for her diploma thesis on the subject »Strategic Management in Statutory Health Insurance Funds«. During her studies she worked for Siemens AG in the industry sector including a six-month internship in Singapore. After her graduation, Anne-Katrin completed an internship at the Institute of Empirical Health Economics before she started working for TK in October 2010. She is currently a trainee at the Department of Disease Management with a focus on Telemedicine.

Wilm Quentin, Dr med., has been working as a research fellow at the Department of Health Care Management at Technical University Berlin since December 2009. He is a medical doctor and holds an MSc in Health Policy, Planning & Financing from the London School of Hygiene and Tropical Medicine (LSHTM) and the London School of Economics (LSE). He studied medicine and political sciences in Würzburg, Munich, Madrid, Leipzig and Marburg, where he graduated in 2007. His research interests are hospital payment systems in Europe, costing studies, and health insurance systems in low-income countries. Wilm Quentin has published articles on a broad range of subjects ranging from »costs of HIV/AIDS-related health services in Rwanda« over »cost-of-illness of dementia« to »hospital payment in Germany«.

David Scheller-Kreinsen, MPP, is research fellow and PhD candidate at the Department for Health Care Management at the Technical University (TU) of Berlin. He studied public policy, economics, political science and industrial relations at the Hertie School of Governance (Berlin), Georgetown University, and the London School of Economics (LSE). David was fellow of the »Studienkolleg zu Berlin« (2005–2006), scholar of the German National Merit Foundation (2003–2007), and was awarded the Elizabeth Thurley Prize by the Industrial Relations Department at the LSE. He conducts research on provider payment systems, hospital cost and quality in Europe. David is Managing Editor of the journal »Health Policy«.

Dr Judith Smith, Head of Policy, is an experienced health services researcher and policy analyst who has studied health care organisation and management in the UK and internationally.
Before joining The Nuffield Trust in February 2009, Judith was based at the Health Services Management Centre, University of Birmingham for 14 years, where she carried out a programme of research and teaching on health commissioning and purchasing; the organisation and management of primary care; health management and leadership; and international health policy. For a number of years, Judith was director of the academic consortium providing the masters education programme for the NHS Graduate Management Training Scheme. Over the period 2007–2009, Judith spent two years working in New Zealand, based at the Health Services Research Centre, Victoria University of Wellington. Judith's research and policy analysis focused on evaluating the implementation and progress of major reforms of primary care in New Zealand. These reforms, set out in the Primary Health Care Strategy, have sought to reduce the cost of fees paid by patients when going to see their GP, as well as seeking to bring about significant changes to the ways in which general practice and other primary care services are organised and delivered within local communities. The publication of three new research reports authored by Judith and other colleagues at the Victoria University of Wellington assess progress to date with implementation of these reforms and have been cited in a recent speech by the New Zealand Minister of Health, when announcing a new phase of primary care development. Judith has published widely, including a book (with Nick Goodwin, 2006) exploring the international move towards more organised or managed primary care, and a textbook designed for health policy makers and managers Healthcare Management (with Kieran Walshe, 2006). She has recently completed her PhD thesis that explored the role of chief executives of health care organisations, with specific reference to the experience of women chief executives.

Dr Frank Verheyen is currently Head of the TK's Scientific Institute for Benefit and Efficiency in Health Care. He received his pharmacy degree from the Westfälische Wilhelms University, Münster, and a PhD in Pharmacoepidemiology/Social Pharmacy from the Humboldt University in Berlin. Additionally, he holds a postgraduate degree in Health Economics from the European Business School, Oestrich Winkel. He started his career as a community pharmacist and started work at The Centre for Drug Information & Pharmacy Practice, being responsible for the development and implementation of pharmaceutical care programmes, in 1997. He joined TK in 2001 as a personal adviser to the Director of the Board of Management. The following years he held several other posts, e.g. project leader »Disease Management Programmes«, Head of the Department of Medicines and Medicines Management.

Dr Caroline Wagner completed her degree in Business Economics at the University of Hamburg. After having worked in marketing for the Northern Association of Company Health Insurance Funds she completed her Master of Science specialised in the Economic History of the European Community at the London School of Economics and Political Science (LSE). Then she received her PhD at the John F. Kennedy Institute of the »Freie Universität« in Berlin. She became a scientific health policy advisor at the Hamburg parliament. After that Caroline Wagner started to work in Strategic Business Development at the statutory health insurance fund »Techniker Krankenkasse« (TK). Since then she has been developing and organising projects concerning the European health care market and EU cross-border care, European health policy as well as comparative cross-country best practice exchange between health systems. Since 2009 she has been researcher and project leader at the »Scientific Institute of TK for Benefit and Efficiency in Health Care« (WINEG) in this field.